The Child Code

The
Child
Code

**The Science Behind Your Child's
True Nature and How to Nurture It**

Dr Danielle Dick

✔ermilion
LONDON

1

Vermilion, an imprint of Ebury Publishing,
20 Vauxhall Bridge Road,
London SW1V 2SA

Vermilion is part of the Penguin Random House group of companies
whose addresses can be found at global.penguinrandomhouse.com

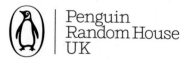

First published in the United Kingdom by Vermilion in 2021
First published in the United States in 2021 by Avery, an imprint of Random House,
a division of Penguin Random House LLC, New York

www.penguin.co.uk

A CIP catalogue record for this book is available from the British Library

ISBN 9781785043475

Printed and bound in Great Britain by Clays Ltd, Elcograf S.p.A.

The authorised representative in the EEA is Penguin Random House Ireland,
Morrison Chambers, 32 Nassau Street, Dublin D02 YH68

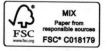

For Aidan

CONTENTS

CONTENTS

AUTHOR'S NOTE

In an effort to make the research accessible, I have necessarily simplified some complex scientific literature. There will be academic colleagues who will surely think that I have oversimplified parts, but I have done my best to balance content and accuracy with readability and applicability. Throughout the book, I provide select scientific references for those who want to dive more into the research literature. For parents who want additional information, I also invite you to visit my website at danielledick.com. Finally, I provide additional recommended readings at the end of the book.

The surveys included in this book are intended to help you better understand your child. They are based loosely on items that are used to assess temperament and personality by researchers. These surveys, however, are not intended to provide formal diagnoses. None of the information in this book should be considered a substitute for professional clinical advice. Guidance for finding a mental health professional can be found in chapter 8.

The Child Code

· · · ▬▬▬ · · ·

Understanding the Child Code

*Before I got married I had six theories about bringing up children;
now I have six children and no theories.*

—John Wilmot (1647–1680)

Close your eyes and imagine your child.

No, not the small person refusing to do homework. Or the one who threw a tantrum at the table because the pasta shapes were butterflies rather than macaroni.

The child you imagined.

Before you had children.

That child was probably a sweet, peaceful baby snuggled up in your arms. An adorable toddler, head thrown back in laughter as you push them on a swing. Maybe they were going to grow up to be a star athlete or the smartest in their class. Maybe you dreamed of a university graduation or a wedding day, a blushing bride or a handsome groom. Point being, we all had ideas of who we wanted our children to be.

But the day-to-day of parenting is less about dreams and more about daily battles. Shoes that your child refuses to put on, precluding you from even making it out the door to the park. Sulking at the dinner table. That fun family trip? Four hours of your child kicking the back of your seat and telling you they don't want to go.

Why is it so hard to shape our children into the dreamy human beings we imagined?

There's certainly no shortage of advice for parents. There are parenting classes, parenting blogs, parenting podcasts, parenting magazines, parenting books, parenting workshops. There are your mother-in-law's ideas about how to handle discipline, and your best friend's tips for sleep training. The overwhelming amount of information is staggering enough, but even worse—much of it conflicts! Human beings have been raising children for millennia; how can it be that we don't have this figured out? The more important question for you as a parent is how to sort through often contradictory guidance to decide what is best.

Why is parenting so darn hard?

It turns out there is a simple answer to that question. The reason parenting is so challenging is that all of that well-meaning advice from your parents and friends and healthcare professionals ignores one of the biggest factors that affects child development: genes.

Our secondary school biology classes didn't give us the full story. DNA doesn't just code for brown or blue eyes, for curly or straight hair; it codes for our brains and our most basic outlook on life. It lays the foundation for our individual temperaments, our natural tendencies, and the unique way each of us interacts with the world. Given the profound influence of genetics on individual behaviour and development, there is no such thing as the "right way" to parent. There is only the "right way" to parent each individual child, and it's only by understanding your child's genetically shaped proclivities that you can guide your child towards becoming his or her best self *and* reduce the daily battles.

The Child Code is about how to figure out that "right way" for *your* child, based on their unique genetic make-up. It's about reducing your stress by helping you cut through piles of information to figure out what really matters (and what doesn't). I'm a scientist who studies genetics and child behaviour, and, more importantly, I'm a parent. I've been in the trenches, and it was my knowledge of the research behind what really influences human behaviour that saved my sanity. I wrote

The Child Code to share this knowledge and to help make your life easier too.

The Illusion of the Super-Parent

Never in the course of human history have we spent so much time trying to actively shape our children. And this high investment in parenting is coming at a tremendous cost, with sharp declines in happiness in couples, and growing rates of anxiety in kids who feel pressured at best, and at worst, under constant assault. The days of our children exploring the woods or roaming the neighbourhood freely, with the only directive being to make it home before dark, are long gone. These days, sending your child to the park unsupervised could end with the police at your doorstep. In some circles, the idea of kids doing their homework unsupervised or taking a standardised test without prep courses would be considered neglectful.

We have allowed the world to make an incredible number of demands on parents, and we have internalised those demands: your decisions are make-or-break! Your every action is critical to whether your child grows up to be well socialised and resilient . . . or a miserable tyrant! If you love your child, you will mould him or her into a successful adult by being the class rep parent, the soccer mum/coach, the PTA president, the Sunday school teacher (and if you *really* love your child, you will ideally be all of these things).

At times, even we parents make it harder on one another. I confess that I have been guilty of this. It's something I bet we have all done at one point or another: seen the toddler throwing a fit at the supermarket, the small child running wild at church, the insolent teenager back-talking to their parent. We have looked from those children to their parents, *and we have judged*. We have said to ourselves: that parent needs to get that child under control! Those parents need to [insert your favourite parenting advice here].

For the first fifteen months of my son's life, I was convinced I had this whole parenting thing figured out. My baby slept for long stretches of time. He cried only when he needed something and he was easily soothed. I remember wondering why people complained about how hard it was to have a newborn. Sure, as someone who was fanatical about getting enough sleep, I found it annoying to have to get up *once* in the night to feed. But that hardly seemed worth all the whining one hears about sleep deprivation in new parents. I had read my books, taken my parenting classes, and my son was pure joy. What was so hard about parenting?

What I didn't appreciate back then was that it wasn't my stellar parenting that led to my happy, sleeping baby. I had just lucked out. What was really driving my child's easy behaviour as an infant was *my child*. Even as a scientist who studies genetics and child behaviour, I had fallen prey to the myth that parenting—for better or worse—is all about the parent. Which is a potent delusion, especially when your child is doing well. It's easy to take credit; it's easy to believe that your child's fabulousness is a reflection of your superior effort. But what if your infant is a sleepless tormentor in the middle of the night? Or your daughter's "terrible twos" begin at six months (and last until she's sixteen)? Are you responsible for that as well? Do you need to read more books, or take more advice from your mother-in-law? When children are struggling, exasperated parents often start to blame themselves or wonder what they are doing wrong. But the research suggests that children's behaviour is driven less by their parents, and more from within.

In the early 1930s, a researcher named Mary Shirley intensively observed twenty-five infants over the first two years of their lives. She started her study interested in infant motor and cognitive development, but what struck her most from following the babies was what she called the "personality nucleus". Based on her observations of the babies across time, she noticed that differences in personality showed up early after birth, with the babies differing systematically on things like irritability, crying, activity levels, and reactions to new people and situations.

Further, these differences appeared to be consistent across different settings and across time. Children who cried a lot, cried whether they were being observed at home or in the infant lab. Children who were highly active were active whether they were at home or in the unfamiliar setting of the lab. Most notably, the differences observed in the children's behaviour didn't seem to be strongly influenced by anything the parent (back in those days, mostly the mother) was doing.

Unique from the Start

The reality is that to a surprisingly large extent, when it comes to your child's behaviour, a great deal is put in place at the moment of conception, when the mother's genes first meet up with the father's, mixing and matching to create an utterly unique human being. And as any parent of more than one child knows, every baby is different, and different from day one. Sure, there are a lot of commonalities. Babies all sleep (probably not as much as you'd like), and poo (probably more than you'd like), and cry and feed. But beyond that, each child is born with his or her own way of being a child, with differences evident from the very beginning.

Developmental psychologists refer to this behavioural distinctiveness as *temperament*, and it is imbedded in the genes, those little strands of information in the nucleus of each cell, which are passed along from the parents to the child. That doesn't mean you can't influence your child's behaviour, simply that you need to realise your influence is constrained—meaning that whatever you do, you have to work with the hand you are dealt. More importantly, if you want to have any hope of success in influencing your child towards one kind of behaviour and away from another, you absolutely have to take their genetic constitution into account.

Genetic differences cause children to differ from the very beginning in *how much they react* to the world (how upset or pleased they are by the things that they encounter), and in *how they regulate* their responses. If they don't want pureed peas, do they throw the dish across the room or simply make a face while obligingly (if unhappily) swallowing? If they see a cute puppy while out in their pram, do they scream with such excitement that you absolutely must stop and play with it? Or do they cower behind your leg, overwhelmed with fear?

What makes temperament especially important for parents is that it is highly stable.

In studies that follow kids across time, fear in infants, measured as early as three months, predicted fear at seven years of age. Anger in infants predicted anger in young children. Highly sociable babies grow up to be highly sociable children and adolescents. Identical twins can be separated at birth and raised by different families and they still turn out to be very similar. Genetics plays a powerful role in shaping how we move through the world.

As you might expect, temperamental characteristics, while stable throughout life, manifest themselves in different ways as children grow. High sociability in a baby shows up as cooing and interacting with other infants and smiling at adults; high sociability in adolescence is the teenager who would rather be at a party than home reading a book or watching a movie with a best friend. The fearful toddler has to be coaxed to try new toys or to climb up on a swing set; the fearful adolescent has to be coaxed to take a part in the school play or to go on the senior trip.

My highly impulsive little boy was the one jumping down from the tops of high trees as a small child, and later asking when he can get a motorcycle and drink beer (sigh, he was only eleven). He does come by these preferences naturally enough—his father is a fighter pilot. Turns out that adventure-seeking and risk-taking are strongly influenced by genetics!

At this point, if you have a happy, sociable small child, you may be feeling all set, and those of you who have highly fearful or irritable little kiddos in your life may be worried.

Don't be. An important thing to remember is that temperamental characteristics are not, in and of themselves, good or bad. The idea of having a sociable, smiling, happy infant may sound very appealing. And smiling, laughing babies, who are open to approaching new toys, new

people, and new situations, are more likely to grow into more extraverted*
adolescents and adults, with all the positive connotations that we associate with being more outgoing. But sociable, active babies are also more
likely to have later problems with control, to be more impulsive, and to
become more frustrated when they don't get their way. They are more
likely to experiment with alcohol in adolescence and to engage in other
risk-taking behaviours with their friends.

By contrast, while a fearful baby may cause parental concern early
on (sometimes even a bit of embarrassment), being more fearful is also
associated with lower impulsivity and aggression. Fearful children are
less likely to get into fights or do the myriad reckless things that adolescents tend to do when they're old enough to be out and about on their
own. But fearful kids are also more prone to sadness and depression.

The point being there is no such thing as a "good" disposition or a "bad"
disposition. There are merely distinctly different, genetically influenced
dispositions, and each of them has its pluses and minuses. How easy or
frustrating different temperamental characteristics are for parents also
can change across a child's developmental stages. Your headstrong toddler may make you want to pull your hair out, but when those same
qualities lead them to stand up against injustice as a young adult, your
heart will swell with pride.

Because temperamental characteristics are not only stable, but associated with different challenges and life outcomes, it is vitally important to understand *your own child's* genetically influenced disposition.
Which is another way of saying that there's no such thing as "one size
fits all" parenting. You have to parent to your child's unique genetic code.

---

* The term "extraverted" has its roots in the Latin word *extra*, meaning "outside", as
compared with "introversion", which is based on the Latin *intro*, meaning "inside". These
terms were introduced by Carl Jung, who believed that extraverts turn their attention
outwards, whereas introverts focus inwards. Accordingly, in the research literature, extraversion is always spelled with an "a", although in the popular press it is often spelled
extroversion. We use the research spelling of *extraversion* throughout this book.

We should also acknowledge up front that some children are more challenging to raise than others. We recognise that simple fact when it comes to parenting a child with autism, or with Down's syndrome. But children who are born with certain dispositional characteristics are also incredibly challenging in unexpected ways that can be really hard on parents. By understanding that basic reality, we can alleviate part of the burden those parents experience, and better support our friends with challenging children.

In medicine today, doctors are working towards individualised therapies formulated to a person's genetic make-up. This is called *precision medicine*, or, alternatively, *personalised medicine*. The idea is that every person's health profile is different; some of us are more predisposed to cancers, others to heart disease, and yet others to substance use or mental health challenges. Some medicines work well for some people, but can be harmful for others. By understanding each person's unique genetic code, doctors can know how best to prevent problems, and to treat them if they do arise.

The same idea applies to parenting. Our children differ in their natural strengths and weaknesses. Being aware of what your child is most likely to enjoy, what they are likely to be good at, what is likely to create challenges for them, and what they are likely to be at risk for, can help you figure out where to focus your efforts as a parent, what parenting strategies are likely to be most effective, and which ones might be harmful. What worked for your first child may not work for your second, and what works for your friend's child may not work for yours.

This is why I hate the term *parenting*. That might sound like a strange thing for a developmental psychologist to say, but the problem with calling what we do as parents *parenting* is that it implies that it is all about the parent. This ignores the other critical factor in the equation—the child! Good parenting is as much about the child as it is about the parent. In the same way that medicine is moving towards individualised care, we're long overdue to embrace a personalised approach to parenting.

Admittedly, it took me a while to adopt this attitude in my own parenting. This was particularly evident when it came to potty training my son. At his day-care centre, mastery of the potty was a requirement for moving up to the three-year-old preschool class. His third birthday came and went, and still he had no interest in being a "big boy"; he seemed perfectly content to stick with nappies and hang out with the two-year-olds. "M&Ms!" my friends told me. "You need to give him M&Ms as a reward for using the potty". So I introduced this inducement, and oh, he wanted the M&Ms all right . . . but he was completely unwilling to use the potty to get them. We simply had regular battles now over why he couldn't have M&Ms when he knew that I had them right there in the cupboard!

Another well-meaning friend came in with her own advice: you have to find his "metric"—figure out what he loves and use that as a reward. For her daughter, it had been picking out what dress to wear. Using the potty meant having a fashion turn. No potty, no special dress. Apparently, it worked like a charm. But when I attempted to implement this technique, it became obvious that my child would rather go to day care naked than use the potty.

After weeks of turmoil and tears (mostly mine), it occurred to me— what my child valued above all else was *winning*, getting his way. Potty training had turned into an all-out battle of wills in our home. Because he felt that I was trying to force this on him, he was just as forcefully refusing. Once I recognised this dynamic, I eased up. I quit talking about potty training, and our daily routine moved on. And you know what happened? Within a couple of weeks (and I'm sure with some encouragement from the no-nonsense day-care provider who was tired of changing his nappies), he just starting using the potty on his own. And off to the three-year-old preschool class he went.

If only I'd wised up sooner and given more attention to what I knew about my son's wilful disposition—particularly his powerful desire to win—I could have saved us both a lot of consternation. Research suggests that kids who are more reactive to punishment (that's definitely my son) are also more sensitive to their parents' requirements for compliance. In other words, the harder you push, the harder they push back. The researchers found, however, that when parents used strategies that de-emphasised power, the child was far more likely to comply. In hindsight, I can see that I was too concerned that (gasp!) my son was two months past his third birthday and still not potty trained. It sent me into over-drive to push him and "fix" the problem, without stepping back to realise how he'd react. You'd think that, as a college professor, I would have taken comfort in the fact that I've never seen a child arrive on campus who isn't potty trained. Eventually, they all figure it out.

Your Child's DNA

Before we talk more about our role as parents, let's talk about where your child's genetic predisposition comes from in the first place. Flash back to basic biology class. No, not the day you dissected a frog, but the day you talked about eggs and sperm and how they come together to form a zygote, which then proceeds to divide and grow until it forms a tiny human being.

DNA is composed of chemicals that line up like the ones and zeros of computer code to form genes, which create the recipe for proteins, which are responsible for all our bodies' processes, from blood pressure to be-haviour. We each consist of a random subset of 50 per cent genetic mate-rial (DNA) from our biological mother, and 50 per cent genetic material (DNA) from our biological father, which mix and match to make each unique child. The 50 per cent each child inherits from each parent is random, and different for each child, which is why your child might have some traits that seem to more closely resemble you and some that more closely resemble their other parent. Every combination of random halves from each parent is what makes your child different from all other human beings, including his or her biological siblings, who also have their own unique combinations of 50/50 subsets of the parents' DNA.

Siblings are generally more similar to each other than two randomly selected people because the subsets of genetic variants they inherited were drawn from the same genetic pool. So siblings share, on average, 50 per cent of their genetic material. But with the human genome consisting of three billion units of DNA, that leaves a lot of room for different combinations, even among full siblings! And with 7.6 billion people currently on the planet, the number of variations is dizzying. Depending on your child's unique mix of genetic variants, they may seem like a mini-you, or leave you wondering if there was a mix-up at the hospital!

But aside from maybe taking a genetic test during pregnancy to make sure everything is going to be OK, most of us don't give much thought to genetics. There are maternity clothes to buy, and a nursery to decorate, and a gazillion choices to make about cots and car seats and prams.

And, of course, there are the parenting classes. Most healthcare professionals don't schedule an initial appointment to confirm a pregnancy until six to eight weeks, but parenting websites recommend that you start taking "prep courses" at nine weeks. There are classes about childbirth, breastfeeding, newborn care, and big-sibling classes. That's followed in the second trimester by prenatal yoga classes, the development of your birthing plan, followed by childbirth education class (which is apparently different from childbirth preparation class). I'm a college professor, and even I think that's a lot of classes!

Admittedly, I took my fair share of parenting classes, and if nothing else, they made me feel more prepared. I was a master swaddler; my child spent most of the first year of his life being wrapped tighter than a burrito at Chipotle. I also did extensive homework on virtually every major and minor decision surrounding my coming bundle of joy.

But all those classes and decisions to prepare for your little one give the illusion of control, which is where "the parenting myth" begins. The books on sleeping and feeding and soothing crying babies suggest that if you do your homework, you'll know how to get your baby to sleep and eat and conform to a schedule. Learn how to do it, implement effectively, and voilà! Happy, healthy baby! Then there's crawling, walking, teething, potty training—a boundless supply of information on how to parent your child through all of their developmental milestones. Somewhere between the point of conception and the birth of that baby, we forget all about the underlying biology—the fact that so much about how your individual child navigates life is a function of what's coded in those genes.

But think about what's going on while you're taking part in all those parenting classes. That baby is growing and developing, *basically without your direction*. Their genetic code is directing their development—arms, legs, fingers and toes, internal organs, brain—all without any conscious input from either parent. It's natural to focus on the things we can control, like picking out a cot and a car seat. But it's critical to remember that while we're decorating the nursery and learning to swaddle, the really important stuff related to child development is happening largely without parental input. It's encoded in our child's DNA.

Which is not to say that the environment you provide isn't important. Extracted DNA sequences in the lab do not spontaneously generate human beings. That little DNA code needs you, and you can do a lot to help it along: good prenatal nutrition, a healthy lifestyle, and low levels of stress are all important for a developing foetus. Conversely, exposure to drugs and environmental toxins can have serious adverse effects on foetal development. As a parent, you of course want to do everything you can to provide the best possible environment for your baby's development. As a mother, you eat healthfully, you take your vitamins, you get exercise. If you're a significant other, you can provide a loving, supportive, stress-free environment for your pregnant partner.

During pregnancy, we realise there's only so much we can do, only so much under our control. Our baby grows and we marvel at that growth. But once that baby pops out (with apologies to all my mother friends who remind me that the birthing process entails a good bit more than popping out), we somehow forget that development throughout childhood is similarly guided by genetic factors, and it's those factors we need to take into account in how we parent.

Nurturing Your Child to Fit Their Nature

After hundreds of years of the "nature/nurture" debate, we now know that nature versus nurture was a false dichotomy. It's not a question of "either/or", but "both/and"—an intermingling of influences, with genetics and environment both playing a role in virtually all behavioural outcomes. The problem for parents is that the focus has stayed all on the nurture piece, and the nature side of the equation has not been given its due. Instead, we stress ourselves to unprecedented levels, thinking that more engagement is what's required, when what we need instead is *smarter* engagement.

This challenge (and opportunity) was summed up nicely by E. O. Wilson, an evolutionary biologist who said that genes place a leash on environmental influence, but it's an elastic leash. In other words, genetics is not destiny, meaning there is nothing parents can do, but neither is it something to be disregarded. Children are not blank slates to be written upon by their well-intentioned parents. By recognising who your child truly is—the unique code they were born with—you can use your influence in ways that resonate with their natural tendencies to help them grow into their best possible self.

Using This Book

The first part of *The Child Code* is about the science behind this fresh approach to parenting. Chapter 1 will introduce you to the research that changed the way we understand what causes human behaviour and revealed the widespread influence of genetics (and limits of parenting) on children's behaviour. (If you don't care much about the research and are willing to take my word for it, you can skip this chapter.) Chapter 2 will help you appreciate how your child's genetic code shapes their development, their personality, their behaviour, and the way they interact with the world. It will help you understand why it matters so much to understand their genetic disposition if you want to be a more effective parent— and a far less stressed one! The second part of the book will focus on your child. Surveys for you to complete about your child's behaviour and tendencies will help you assess your child's genetic proclivities. Then, I'll walk you through how to use that information to adapt your parenting to your specific child, to help them reach their potential and avoid pitfalls. And most importantly, we'll talk about how to relax and draw confidence with this information for happier parenting. So, let's get started!

Takeaways

- Your child's genes play a central role in shaping their brain and behaviour.

- Parenting advice is often conflicting because it ignores the important role of each child's genetic make-up in influencing their behaviour. This is why what works for one child may not work for another.

- Understanding your child's genetic make-up can help you parent your unique child, supporting them to reach their potential and overcome natural challenges. In addition, it will create a more harmonious relationship with your child, and reduce parenting stress.

PART 1

Everything You Need to Know
About the Science of Human Behaviour
(and Nothing More)

CHAPTER 1

Nature versus Nurture:
The Science Is In

Let's start at the beginning: where did the ingrained idea that parents play such a critical role in shaping child behaviour come from?

The widespread emphasis on (and misunderstanding of) the role of parents can be traced back to the origins of the field of child psychology. As a parent you spend a lot of time trying to understand your child's behaviour, but researchers have been trying to understand children for *hundreds* of years. In 1787, German philosopher Dietrich Tiedemann published the first account of child development, recording his son's behaviour across the first thirty months of his life. Tiedemann was deeply influenced by the English philosopher John Locke, who lived in the 1600s and believed that we all start life as blank slates, with our development entirely determined through our experiences. Nearly a hundred years later, *The Mind of the Child* (1882) was published by Wilhelm Preyer, another German professor. It described the development of his own daughter over her first few years of life, and is frequently cited as the beginning of modern-day child psychology.

From these early "baby biographies", which recounted observations of a single child growing up, the field expanded to include studies of small numbers of children who were observed extensively across development. Over time, these studies began to include the children's parents as well, as developmental psychologists became interested in the role of parenting. Across this evolution, a consistent, central feature of child development research remained, namely, that the field has been based on *observational* studies. But this design feature has a massive limitation, and is at the heart of why there is so much pressure placed on parents when it comes to their children's behaviour.

The Traditional Family Study—And Its Limitations

It seems intuitive that if you want to understand the influence of parents on their children, you would (drumroll) study parents and their children. By now, there have been thousands of studies of parents and children conducted, and these studies form the basis for most of the child-rearing advice that's out there. In these studies, researchers ask parents to report on their parenting practices, and they measure children on a particular outcome. Sometimes they ask children to report on their parents and on themselves; sometimes they ask the parents to report on themselves and their children. And sometimes researchers get information from other reporters as well, such as teachers or other caregivers.

These studies consistently find correlations (a statistical measure of similarity) between aspects of parenting and outcomes in children, and these findings are usually interpreted as evidence for the role of parents in shaping children's behaviour.

For example, a consistent finding is that positive parenting practices, such as parental warmth and parental involvement, are associated with fewer emotional and behavioural problems in children. Conversely, harsh or inconsistent parenting is associated with more behaviour problems in children. Voilà! Proof for the importance of parenting, right?

Not so fast.

There are lots of good reasons to treat your child with warmth, and to practise consistent, positive parenting. But the problem with these studies is that they are often (mis)interpreted to mean that the parenting behaviour is *causing* the child behaviour.

But there's a flaw in that logic. It boils down to the basic principle we all learned in secondary school science class: correlation does not equal causation. In other words, just because two things are related does not mean that one caused the other.

The best way to make causal attributions is with a controlled experiment. Child psychologists are at a disadvantage because they can't experimentally assign children to different parents. If we could randomly assign children to grow up with (for example) parents with fewer rules, and parents with stricter rules, that would allow us to test whether differences in parenting rules are related to differences in children's outcomes. Random assignment to parents would mean that many different types of children get assigned to the few rules and strict rules groups, so we can more definitively conclude that any differences found between the groups are due to the difference in parenting. Randomised experimental designs are what we use to assess whether interventions or new pharmaceuticals are effective.

But correlations, like those we observe between parents and children, don't tell us anything about causality, because they are not informative about the direction of the effect. *Maybe* when parents treat their children with warmth, they behave better. *Maybe* when parents are harsh with their children, those children become more aggressive. But it's equally plausible that children who are better behaved invoke more warmth from their parents. When my child compliantly pulls on his clothes and is ready and waiting by the door to head to school, I'm much warmer than when he sulks in bed and refuses to get up. It's far easier to be loving towards a child who is behaving delightfully than one who is throwing a tantrum! The same logic applies to misbehaviour: it's equally possible that the child who is more aggressive is actually causing the parents to respond with harsher discipline in an effort to improve the child's behaviour. Maybe those parents would have been warm and delightful if their child wasn't acting out. The bottom line is that when we find a correlation between a parenting practice and a child outcome, we can't know which of these possibilities is the correct one. Is the parenting causing the child's behaviour or is the child's behaviour driving the parenting?

It turns out this is a very important distinction. The misinterpretation of parent–child correlations as evidence for the causal role of parenting has had profound consequences. A particularly striking example can be found in the way we have viewed autism over time. Autism was originally thought to be caused by cold mothers who didn't socialise their babies properly. Medical professionals came to this conclusion after studies showed that mothers of children who developed autism were less likely to smile and coo and interact with their infants in typical mum ways. There was a correlation between mothers' lack of interaction with their babies and autism. The researchers incorrectly concluded that cold mothering was *causing* the children to develop autism. What researchers eventually discovered when they studied those families across time was that mothers of children who later developed autism started out exactly like mothers of children who didn't develop problems. But children who went on to develop autism didn't respond to those maternal cues in the way that most typically developing babies do—the babies didn't coo, or maintain eye contact with the mother, or seem to enjoy the interaction. So over time the mums did less of it. It wasn't the mother's behaviour influencing the child's outcome at all—it was the child's behaviour that influenced the mum.

Studying children and parents across time is one way to start to tease apart the direction of the effect, because you can examine whether parental behaviour influences future child behaviour after taking into account what the child was like to begin with, and vice versa. And when researchers study parents and children across time, they find something surprising. Child behaviour generally has a stronger influence on future parenting than parenting behaviour has on future child behaviour. In other words, our children shape our parenting more than our parenting shapes our children.

For example, a large study led by several prominent child development colleagues has followed nearly 1,300 children and their parents across nine countries, representing twelve cultural groups around the world (China, Colombia, Italy, Jordan, Kenya, the Philippines, Sweden, Thailand, and the United States). They studied the families when the children were ages eight, nine, ten, twelve, and thirteen, and tested for bidirectional influences between parenting behaviour and children's emotional and behavioural problems across time. They found that, across all cultural groups, children had large effects on subsequent parenting: more emotional or behavioural challenges in children predicted less parental warmth and more parental control at the next age, even after taking into account previous child and parent behaviour. Conversely, there was little evidence that parenting predicted future child behaviour. The degree to which parents were warm or controlling did not have a significant effect on the likelihood that children would have emotional or behavioural problems in the future. The study emphasised how children drive future parenting, as parents react to their children's behaviour, more so than parents are able to shape future child behaviour—a finding that was consistent around the globe.

There's another problem with interpreting parent–child correlations to mean that the parent's behaviour is *causing* the child's behaviour, or vice versa. It could be something else altogether influencing both the child's and parent's behaviour and making them look similar, even if the behaviours are not directly influencing one another. We call this a *third variable*. Think about this example: there is a correlation between buying ice cream and wearing sunglasses. Does that mean that ice cream eating makes people put on sunglasses? Or that wearing sunglasses makes people eat ice cream? Of course not; the reason that eating ice cream and wearing sunglasses is correlated is because there's something else influencing both behaviours—there's a third variable at play: warm, sunny days. Warm, sunny days lead people to be more likely to eat ice cream *and* to wear sunglasses. In the case of correlations between biological parents and their children, that something else—that other thing that could be causing the behaviour both in the parent and the child—is their shared genes.

Returning to our examples above, we know that behavioural and emotional problems are genetically influenced. So when we find that parental warmth is associated with positive outcomes in children, there are three possible interpretations: (1) parental warmth leads kids to behave better; (2) well-behaved kids lead parents to be warmer towards them; or (3) the correlation is purely a by-product of the fact that genes influence emotions and behaviour, and biological parents and children share their genes. So, for example, parents who carry genes that influence good behaviour (making them more likely to be positive, warm parents) are more likely to pass along a higher genetic propensity towards good behaviour to their children. We also know that aggression is genetically influenced, so the fact that parental harsh discipline is correlated with increased aggression could be because (1) parental harsh discipline causes child aggression; (2) child aggression causes their parents to discipline them more harshly; or (3) parents who discipline harshly are more likely to carry aggression-related genes, and their child is accordingly more likely to carry genes that make them more aggressive. These possibilities aren't mutually exclusive; in actuality, all of these processes, or some combination thereof, could be going on. (Remember that your kids get a random mix of only 50 per cent of your DNA, and 50 per cent of their other parent's DNA, which is why there is no guarantee that your kids will inherit all your fabulous—or least desirable—characteristics.)

In short, when we see correlations between parenting practices and child outcomes, it's tempting to conclude that parents are influencing their children (and lots of child "experts" do this!), but it's equally likely that the children are driving their parents' behaviour, or that the similarities between parents and children are simply due to their shared genetic make-up. Maybe those children would have been just as wonderful, or delinquent, even without their wonderful or delinquent parents. Without an experimental design, we have no way of knowing. We know that something is creating correlations between parenting and children's outcomes; we just don't know what that something is. Fortunately, we have some natural experiments that allow us to separate out the importance of genetic and environmental influences, and to study to what extent the child's genes are driving the behaviour and to what extent parental influence is actually having an impact.

Adoption Studies: The Role of Genes Emerges

The first, and most ideal, "natural experiment" that allows researchers to tease apart genetic and environmental influences is adoption studies. When we were talking about correlations between parents and children (and how they don't allow you to figure out how important parenting actually is), I was referring to *biologically related* parents and children. When parents and children are biologically related, they share both their genes and their home environments, so when they look similar, you can't tell what caused that similarity—was it shared genes or was it family influence? But in adoptive families, genetics and environment get split up. Adopted children (when raised by non-relatives) share genes with parents who are not providing their home environment (their biological parents), and their environments are provided by people who didn't give them their genetic make-up (their adoptive parents). In other words, there is a perfect natural separation of genetic and environmental influences. Genes from biological parents; environment from adoptive parents.

This means that researchers can collect data from adopted children, their biological parents, and their adoptive parents (and sometimes siblings) in order to figure out how much genetic predispositions play a role and how much the family environment matters. Do adopted children act more like their biological parents (which would imply genetic predispositions are important), or do they more closely resemble their adoptive parents (which would imply that environmental influences related to

23

parenting are more important)? This is a natural experiment that separates genetic influence from parental environmental influence.

One of the most powerful examples of how adoption studies shed light on the causes of human behaviour can be found in the case of schizophrenia. Schizophrenia is a severe mental disorder that affects about 1 per cent of the population, with affected individuals experiencing hallucinations and/or delusions. As with autism, doctors originally believed that schizophrenia was caused by bad mothers (mothers get blamed for everything, sigh). In this case, they were called *schizophrenogenic mothers*, and were thought to be cold, detached mothers who provided inadequate emotional attachments for their children, which, the theory went, caused those children to develop schizophrenia. Just think about that for a minute: your child develops a severe disorder in which they lose touch with reality, and if you're the mother, *you are told that it's your fault*. Imagine how awful that must have been—first, to see your child struggling, and then, to add insult to injury, to be told that you were responsible! Unfortunately, this wasn't just the case for schizophrenia (and autism). Until the 1950s, most doctors thought that the vast majority of mental and behavioural health disorders were due to failures on the part of parents. But then along came adoption studies.

In the late 1960s, a researcher published a study in which they followed fifty children who were born to mothers with schizophrenia in Oregon state hospitals between 1915 and 1945. All of the babies had been separated from their mothers within the first few days of life and adopted by parents who did not have schizophrenia. The researchers followed up on the children when they were in their mid thirties, and compared them to adopted children whose biological mothers had no history of schizophrenia. They found that 17 per cent of the children who had biological mothers with schizophrenia still developed the debilitating disorder, despite having no contact with their "schizophrenogenic mother". In other words, nearly one in five of the children who shared genes (but no environment) with a biological parent who had schizophrenia developed the disorder, compared to the general population rate of one in a hundred. None of the comparison children, who did not have a biological mother with schizophrenia, developed the disorder. This was the first powerful evidence that genes were important in the development of schizophrenia; it wasn't actually bad parenting at all that caused the disorder. We now know that schizophrenia is a highly genetically influenced disorder, with a heritability of about 80 per cent.

In the case of schizophrenia, adoption studies made it pretty clear that genetics was responsible, not parenting. But it's not just severe disorders like schizophrenia that show the role of biology. Virtually all outcomes that have been studied using the adoption design—ranging from alcohol problems to infant shyness—have yielded unambiguous evidence of genetic effects. Children resemble their biological parents for all kinds of behavioural outcomes, *even when they aren't raised by them!* Our genetic programming is powerful stuff.

But, parents, don't despair—your child's destiny is not *all* about their genes. Adoption studies have also been pivotal in pointing to the role of the home environment. As one example, a Swedish adoption study examined criminal behaviour. What makes some kids more likely to get in trouble with the law?* Sweden has been home to some of the biggest adoption studies in the world because it has population-based registries that provide information on family relationships, including births and adoptions, for all individuals born or living in Sweden. It is possible to link this family information to a host of other national registries, ranging from health records, to hospitalisations, to prescription medication registries, to criminal records. (Americans are always taken aback when I talk about the research we are able to do in the Nordic countries as a result of their national registries; it's a very different cultural mentality in which the society places a high value on contributing to

---

* In the United States, there are forces like systemic racism that profoundly shape criminal justice system involvement. Sweden is a more homogeneous country that does not have these same challenges, which makes it possible to do a less biased study of the factors that contribute to criminal justice system involvement.

research.) These national databases make it possible to investigate how similar adopted children are to their biological parents and how similar they are to their adoptive parents, on any of the outcomes that are tracked in the national population-based registers.

In order to better understand what factors influenced antisocial behaviour, researchers collected information about criminal convictions from the Swedish Crime Register in adopted children, their biological parents, and their adoptive parents. They found that adopted children who had biological parents with criminal records also showed elevated rates of criminal behaviour, even though they were not raised by those parents. While there is no gene for criminal behaviour, remember from the introduction that traits like aggression and impulsivity show up early in life as fairly stable, genetically influenced temperamental factors, and of course these characteristics are related to the likelihood of getting in trouble with the law.

Importantly, the researchers conducting this adoption study also created an "environmental risk score" based on whether the *adoptive* parents and siblings had criminal convictions, as well as whether there was a divorce, death, or medical illness in the adoptive family, with the presumption that these would be environmental stressors. It turns out that environmental risk was also associated with elevated rates of criminal behaviour in the adopted children. In other words, there was evidence that both genes *and* home environment mattered when it comes to criminal behaviour in kids.

Adoption studies provide an important theoretical separation of genes and environments, but they have their limitations. Adoptions are increasingly "open", whereby adoptees have some continued contact with biological parents. This interferes with the natural separation of genes-but-no-environment from biological parents, environment-but-no-genes from adoptive parents. Another complicating factor is that the prenatal environment of adopted children is provided by their biological mother, so you can't disentangle prenatal environmental effects from the genetic effects; you can only study environmental effects that start when the children are placed into their adoptive homes after birth. Perhaps one of the biggest challenges with doing adoption studies these days is that in many parts of the world adoptions are becoming increasingly rare, in part due to decreased stigma surrounding pregnancy outside of marriage. This makes it more challenging to conduct adoption studies outside the information that can be obtained from large national registry studies, such as the one in Sweden, which are limited to studying outcomes that can be obtained from government databases.

Twin Studies:
A Powerful Way to Understand Genetic Influence

Fortunately, there's another natural experiment that allows us to study how important genetic and environmental influences are: twin studies. And while adoption studies are becoming more difficult to conduct, twins are becoming increasingly common. Twins are interesting in all kinds of ways. Imagine having a carbon copy of yourself walking around the planet! That's your reality if you are an identical twin. Twins essentially come in two flavours, which are commonly called *identical twins* and *fraternal twins*. Identical twins result when a single egg is fertilised by a single sperm, but at some point during cell division, for reasons that are still not fully understood, the zygote splits into two. Voilà! Genetically identical individuals!

Technically, scientists and medical professional don't call them identical twins, they call them *monozygotic* (MZ) twins, *mono* meaning one, referring to the fact that they developed from one zygote. Because MZ twins develop from a single zygote, they share 100 per cent of their genetic material; they have genetically identical DNA sequences. And because they are genetically identical, MZ twins are always of the same sex (either both boys or both girls).

The other type of twins are fraternal twins, or in science speak: *dizygotic* (DZ) twins. These twins are so named because they come from two (*di* being the Greek word for "two") zygotes. Dizygotic twins result from two eggs fertilised by two sperm, just like ordinary siblings, except that fertilisation happens at the same time, so they share an intrauterine environment, and hence are age matched, unlike ordinary siblings. DZ twins share on average 50 per cent of their genetic material, just like ordinary siblings, and accordingly can be of the same sex, or opposite sex, just like any pair of siblings.

Twins provide a natural experiment because they are essentially two "types" of age-matched siblings who are being raised together in the same family, by the same parents, but they differ in how much of their genetic make-up they share. Scientists who do twin research often collect data from thousands of twin pairs—both MZ and DZ—and then compare how similar MZ twins are to each other, as compared to how similar DZ twins are to each other. If something is entirely determined by the home environment, then it shouldn't matter that one type of twins (MZs) shares more genetic material than the other type (DZs); they should be equally similar.

For example, if having a parent with alcohol use disorder causes increased alcohol problems for environmental reasons, perhaps because there are more stressors in the home or exposure to alcohol, then siblings who have parents with an alcohol use disorder should show an elevation in alcohol problems, regardless of how much genetic variation they share. In other words, if you took any two kids and put them in a home with a parent with alcohol problems, if it is all environmental, then they should all show an elevation in alcohol issues. Of course we can't do this ethically, but twins provide a variation on this theme: kids being raised together with the same parents, some of whom share more of their genetic make-up with each other (MZs) than others (DZs).

Then again, if it isn't just all environment, if a person's genetic make-up is important in influencing how at risk they are for an alcohol use disorder (for example), then MZ twins should be more similar on their alcohol outcomes than DZ twins, because they share more similar genes. If something is entirely genetically determined, then we would expect that MZ twins should be exactly alike (a correlation of 1.0), since they share all of their genetic code, and that DZ twins should be half as alike (a correlation of 0.5), since they share only half of their genetic variation. So, to the extent that MZ twins are more alike than DZ twins for any behaviour being studied, it tells us that behaviour is under genetic influence.

Finally, if MZ twins are not exactly alike (they rarely are for most temperamental and behavioural outcomes, which is why scientists don't like calling them "identical" twins), it tells us that there must be other random environmental influences that impact our trait of interest. For example, one twin could experience a life stressor, such as a car accident or a romantic breakup, that the other one didn't. Or one twin might have a different group of friends than his/her co-twin. In short, when MZ twins aren't identical for an outcome being studied, we don't know exactly why the twins are different; we just know that there must be some kind of environmental influences at play that are making them different, since genetically they are identical.

There have now been *thousands* of twin and adoption studies of virtually every behaviour you can imagine. These studies have been carried out by researchers around the world. Many countries have national twin registries based on birth records, such as large-scale studies in Finland, Norway, Denmark, and Sweden. I work on a study of more than ten thousand twins, representing all twins born in Finland over a ten-year period, and we have followed them from age twelve through to mid-adulthood to understand the development of alcohol use problems. There is a large twin registry in the Netherlands that has enrolled around 120,000 twins, with a subset of those twins enrolled as young children and studied, along with their parents, at ages three, five, seven, ten, and twelve years, to provide information about early child behavioural development. Other large twin studies have been created by targeted recruitment of twins, such as twin registries established in several states through driver's licence or birth records. My current university is home to one such twin registry in the mid-Atlantic region of the United States. Using these registries, there have been studies of substance use and psychiatric disorders; studies of personality and intelligence; studies of divorce, happiness, voting behaviour, religiosity, social attitudes, and almost anything else you can think of! Nearly every behaviour has been studied using twin (and/or adoption) designs, in order to figure out to what extent genetic and environmental influences impact that behaviour.

The overarching conclusion from all those studies is that *virtually everything is under genetic influence*. Monozygotic twins (who have identical genetic codes) are almost always more similar than dizygotic twins (who share just half of their genetic code), despite both siblings being raised in the same family, by the same parents. For example, here are illustrative twin correlations from a variety of studies of child behaviour that are representative of the findings twin researchers routinely obtain (recalling that similarity between twins is measured by a correlation, which can range from 0, meaning that the twins' outcomes are completely different, to 1.0, meaning that the twins' behaviour is identical, with higher numbers indicating the twins are more alike): a huge study of self-control found that MZ twins correlated at 0.6, whereas DZ twins had a correlation of 0.3. Anxiety/depression in three-year-olds: for boys, MZs correlate 0.7 and DZs correlate 0.3; for girls, MZs correlate 0.7 and DZs correlate 0.4. Behaviour problems in seven-year-olds for boys, MZs correlate 0.6, DZs correlate 0.4; for girls, MZs correlate 0.6, DZs correlate 0.3. I won't bore you with more numbers. You get the idea. For boys and for girls, for virtually all behaviours studied in children (and adults), MZs are more highly correlated than DZs, meaning that siblings who share more of their genetic code are more similar. Genes matter. We are not born as blank slates. John Locke, the philosopher who influenced the very beginnings of the field of child psychology, was wrong. Children are born with genetic codes that impact whether they are naturally more fearful, or impulsive, or aggressive, or any number of other characteristics.

With such widespread evidence for genetic influences on behaviour, you may wonder: is everything genetic? Once you understand how genes shape so many aspects of our behaviour and lives (which we'll discuss further in the next chapter), it's actually hard to think of things that show no genetic influence. Seriously. Take a moment to try it.

Here's a couple: the first language you speak is entirely environmentally influenced. The reason I started speaking English and not Chinese is not because I was genetically predisposed to speak English. I started speaking English because the people around me spoke English. That's not to say that one's *ability* to learn a language isn't genetically influenced (it is), but which language you start with is all environment. This is also true for initial religious affiliation. You don't become baptised as a Catholic versus an Anglican because of your genetic predisposition. You're born as a Catholic or Anglican (or Methodist, or Buddhist, or Jewish, or . . .) because it's the religious affiliation of your family. That said, the degree to which people report being religious as they get older *is* genetically influenced.

When you go beyond traditional family studies, and use research designs that actually tease apart the influence of our children's genetic make-up from the influence of our parenting, the evidence is clear and compelling: our genes impact our temperaments and tendencies, and all kinds of aspects of our behaviour and our lives. A prominent behaviour geneticist, Dr Eric Turkheimer, at the University of Virginia (coincidentally the professor from whom I took my first psychology class) has famously written that the first law of behaviour genetics is, "All human behavioural traits are heritable". The facts are in. The studies have been done. Of course there are some exceptions to the rule, but overwhelmingly, the evidence shows that human behaviour is incontrovertibly influenced by our genetics.

Separated at Birth: A Case Study in the Power of Genes

Jim Lewis and Jim Springer met at the age of thirty-nine years old. They drove the same kind of car and went on holiday at the same beach in Florida. They both smoked Salem cigarettes. They were both nail biters. They were both married to women named Betty, had divorced women named Linda. One had a son named James Alan; the other's son was named James Allan. Both had pet dogs named Toy. Both were bad at spelling and good at maths. Both did carpentry and had some law enforcement training. Both were six feet tall and 180 pounds. The men had never met before age thirty-nine. Jim and Jim were identical twins separated at birth and raised by different adoptive families, unknown to each other until they were reunited in a research lab after nearly four decades.

MZ twins separated at birth are another variation on the twin design that allows us to understand how important genetic and environmental influences are. People are fascinated by this experimental design. Just imagine: two genetically identical babies placed into different families and raised by separate parents.* It creates a unique opportunity to study how similar or different those genetically identical individuals turn out to be when raised by different sets of parents.

As you might expect, identical twins separated at birth and placed with different (non-related) families are pretty rare. But in the late 1970s, researchers from the University of Minnesota launched a landmark study where they began tracking down twin pairs separated in infancy. Over the course of twenty years, they found more than one hundred pairs of separated twins and brought them into the lab for a week of psychological and physiological assessments. In many cases, it was the first time the twins had ever met. The Jim twins are a famous example of these reunited twin pairs.

The remarkable finding from those studies was that MZ twins raised apart were virtually as similar as MZ twins raised together, on everything from personality and temperament, to social attitudes, to

---

* Note: Of course researchers can't ethically separate twins and place them into different homes without consent. The movie *Three Identical Strangers* (2018) tells the tragic story of an adoption agency that was separating twins unethically and placing them into different families for research purposes.

work-related and leisure-time interests. The shocking finding from this groundbreaking project was that *being raised by the same parents didn't make the siblings any more similar than if they had been raised in different families.*

In Dr Turkheimer's famous paper on the laws of behaviour genetics, the second law, right after "All human behavioural traits are heritable", is "The effect of being raised in the same family is smaller than the effect of genes". The science shows that genetically identical individuals grow up to be remarkably similar, even when raised in totally different families.

The Big Question: Do Parents Matter?

But wait, do these remarkable findings suggest that what kind of parent you are really doesn't make a difference? Unfortunately, this is often how findings from the field of behaviour genetics are interpreted. It is not a message that parents want to hear, so basically the research has been ignored. But sticking our collective heads in the sand and pretending that genes don't have a profound influence on our children's behaviour and outcomes doesn't help anyone. It has led to unprecedented levels of stress in parents, who have doubled down in their parental "shaping" efforts, wondering why they can't get their children to [fill in the blank]. It has led to a culture of judgement in which we are quick to criticise parents whose children are misbehaving, in the belief that the parents must be doing something wrong. And even more importantly, it has meant that we are far less effective parents than we could be if we recognised and understood our children's natural genetic tendencies.

The fact that genes have a profound influence on kids' behaviour doesn't mean that parents don't matter. It just means that genes matter. And that parents matter in different ways than we may have thought. And that's what the next chapter is all about.

Takeaways

- Most of what we are told about parenting comes from family studies finding correlations between parenting practices and children's behaviour. These studies have been misinterpreted to mean that parenting shapes child behaviour, but it is equally possible that the child's behaviour is driving the parenting, or that parents and children are correlated simply due to their shared genes. Because of these fundamental flaws, most family studies actually tell us very little about the effects of parenting.

- Adoption studies allow us to tease apart the effects of genetic predispositions from the effects of the home environment. Adoption studies test how similar children are to their biological parents (with whom they share genes but no environment) as compared to their adoptive parents (who provide parenting but no genes). These studies overwhelmingly find that children resemble their biological parents, providing strong evidence for genetic influences on behaviour.

- Twin studies also allow us to study the relative importance of genetic influences and environmental influences by comparing monozygotic (MZ, or identical) twins, who are genetically identical, to dizygotic (DZ, or fraternal) twins, who share on average just 50 per cent of their genetic material. These studies find that MZ twins are more alike than DZ twins for virtually every behaviour studied, further supporting the importance of genetic influence on human behaviour. Identical twins raised by different families turn out to be about as similar as identical twins raised by the same parents, providing further evidence for the importance of genes on life outcomes.

- Taken together, these studies compellingly show that genetic predispositions play a large role in shaping child behaviour; the influence of genes is bigger than the influence of parenting practices.

CHAPTER 2

It's Complicated: The Ways That Genes Influence Our Lives

I hope that by now I have persuaded you that your child is a fascinating bundle of walking genes. These genes influence how much children talk back, how much they eagerly comply, how much they like to read, how much they cry, and even how much they freak out about the idea of Father Christmas being in their house. Yes, you read that right. My six-year-old niece is terrified of the idea of someone being inside their house, so much so that every Christmas, they write a note to Father Christmas instructing him to stay downstairs (a compromise my sister coaxed her into for the sake of their other child).

Genes have a profound impact on our children's behaviour. But how does that really work in a practical sense?

One of my favourite articles is called "A Gene for Nothing" by Robert Sapolsky, a fellow professor and best-selling author of books with titles like *Why Zebras Don't Get Ulcers*. I love the piece because even though I do genetics research, like Sapolsky, I hate the phrase "gene for". The media, however, love it. Turn on the news and you'll read about the gene for alcoholism! The gene for depression! The gene for breast cancer! The gene for aggression! But the truth is much more complex. Human beings have only about 20,000 genes, and most of them code for things like eyes and ears and arms and arteries. If there was a gene for everything in our biology and our behaviour, we would run out of genes quickly. Fruit flies have about 14,000 genes, and our children are a good bit more complicated than fruit flies, so something else must be going on.

Although single genes with big effects are what we learned about in secondary school biology (remember doing Punnett squares for eye colour?), for those of us who don't have rare single gene disorders, our genetic predispositions affect our lives in subtler ways. There is no gene for sociability, for fear, for temper tantrums so monumental they open a new checkout queue at the supermarket to get you out the door faster.

Instead, complex behaviours, ranging from intelligence to personality, are influenced by lots of genes—probably hundreds or thousands of them. So, for example, your child's genetic tendency towards anxiety (or impulsivity, or fear, or any other behaviour) is a product of which variants they carry across all of those thousands of genes that influence anxiety. Some genetic variants increase risk, others decrease risk, and where your child naturally falls on each behavioural dimension is the sum of all the risk and protective genes they carry that influence that behaviour.

The fact that most complex outcomes are influenced by many, many genes is why on average kids resemble their parents, but not always. A pair of basketball players can have a short child. This is because two really tall people are likely to have more "tall genes" (genes that increase height) than "short" ones (genes that decrease height), which is why they sum up to above-average height. But being tall doesn't mean they don't carry any short genes; they just have fewer of them. Because the 50 per cent of our parents' genetic variants we inherit is random, it can mean that, by chance, a child could get most of their tall parent's short genes. It isn't *likely*, since a tall parent has more tall genes than short ones, but it is *possible*. That's how two tall parents can have a short kid. Two smart parents can have an average-intelligence child. Two extraverts can have an introvert. On average, kids are going to resemble their (biological) parents, but because every child is a roll of the genetic dice (i.e. which 50 per cent of yours and 50 per cent of your partner's genetic variants come together), you never know!

Researchers are still in the process of identifying all of the genes involved in different disorders and outcomes, and though we have found some, we still have a long way to go. Because there is so much variation in behaviour, and people don't naturally fall into distinct groups (e.g. impulsive or not), we know there must be many, many genes involved to create the bell-shaped distribution we observe for most behaviours in the population. These genes don't code "for" a particular behaviour; they influence behaviour by impacting the way our brains form.

Individual differences in brain structure and function are highly heritable, meaning they are strongly influenced by our genes. In turn, the ways our brains are wired contribute to our natural tendencies towards fear, anxiety, frustration, and reward seeking. Our brains influence our attention, memory, cognition, and how we learn. They impact complex processes, like how we read social cues, and basic biological processes, like circadian rhythms and sleep. By influencing our brain development, our genes lay the foundation for the many differences that make each of us unique—in terms of our biology *and* our behaviour.

As an example, in one of the projects I work on, we are trying to understand why some people are more at risk of developing alcohol problems than others. As part of the study, we measure brain wave activity in our participants. We find differences in the brains of individuals with alcohol use disorders. That may seem unsurprising, as you might guess that using a lot of substances changes one's brain (it does). But what's most interesting is that similar differences in brain wave activity are also found in many of the children of parents with alcohol use disorders—*before those children have ever tried alcohol*. The differences reflect brain mechanisms involved in impulsivity, reward processing, and cognitive control. What's more, these brain differences aren't just related to alcohol use disorder; they are also found in children with ADHD, behaviour problems, and other drug problems, all of which are related to impulsivity and self-control. In other words, some children get brains that are wired to make them more impulsive, and this can put them at risk for a variety of different outcomes across development, ranging from ADHD and behaviour problems when they are young, to substance use problems as they get older.

So, our genes influence the unique way that our brains are structured, which influences our behavioural tendencies. But that's only the first step. The other big reason that genetic factors play such an important role in our life outcomes is that in addition to directly impacting our natural tendencies towards certain behaviours, they are also deeply linked to our environment. Through these gene-environment connections, our genes magnify their influence on our behaviour in complicated and indirect ways. It is by understanding these gene–environment pathways through which genetic influences unfold that we can play our biggest role as parents.

Gene–Environment Interplay: A Critical Way That Genes Shape Behaviour

Despite the intensity of the long-running nature versus nurture debate, it actually makes no sense to think about genes *versus* environment. This is because our genes and our environment are not separate "things" that shape us. The genes we inherit may be the luck of the draw, but our environments are not (for the most part) random things that happen to us. Our genetic tendencies influence our exposure to certain environments, how we experience those environments, and the degree to which those environments influence us. Researchers call this intertwining of our genetic predispositions and our environmental experiences *gene–environment correlation*. Simply stated, our genes and our environments are related to one another. And it turns out that our genotypes and our environments are intertwined in all kinds of ways.

Way 1: Evocative and Reactive Gene-Environment Correlation

Meet Anthony. Anthony was a sociable little guy from the time he was a toddler. At age three, he loved to wear his Batman mask and cape at the supermarket. He was prone to running up to strangers and telling them about his superpowers (never mind that Batman didn't actually have any) and asking them about theirs. It was pretty adorable and people smiled and chatted to him. Although it was not intentional, these interactions gave Anthony confidence in talking to adults. He learned (inadvertently) that most adults were friendly, and conversation was fun. When he started preschool, he would linger in the classroom and chat with his teacher. He asked if he could help wipe off the boards at the end of the day so he could spend time with her. The teacher thought Anthony was adorable. Whenever she needed a volunteer, his hand would shoot up. She put him at a desk in the front of the classroom. This had the effect of making Anthony more engaged in his learning, in part because he wanted to please his teacher, and in part because he was front and centre. His grades got a nudge. He established a pattern of positive relations with his teachers. Fast-forward twelve years and Anthony headed off to Harvard and eventually became a rocket scientist. OK, not really, but you get the idea.

Our temperaments and predispositions influence minuscule aspects of our day-to-day lives, and over time these nudges have cumulative effects that add up. Anthony's genetic predisposition nudged him towards a series of "environmental" experiences that further influenced the way he interacted with his environment. Those environmental influences started to add up, and in the story version of his life, eventually took him into space. But those "environmental" effects all started from, and were a by-product of, his genetically influenced temperament.

Our temperaments influence the way we move through the world, and since our temperaments are genetically influenced, this means our genes are driving all kinds of aspects of our day-to-day experiences.

If you are a generally irritable person, you're more likely to be grumpy with the supermarket checkout person, who might just further slow down how quickly (or not) they check you out. This further confirms your view that people are generally annoying and makes you more irritable.

Or maybe you are someone who is prone to anxiety. A new neighbour moves in next door. You think about taking them a welcome gift, but then worry about what to drop off. You could bake them biscuits, but what if they don't eat sweets? You could take them a bottle of wine, but would they be offended if they don't drink alcohol? Maybe you could drop off a lasagna . . . but what if they have dietary restrictions? In the end you take them nothing. Years go by and you never get to know the people living two doors down, other than a friendly wave as you drive by on the street. You've always thought about how nice it would be to know the neighbours better so that you could have someone you felt comfortable borrowing an egg from or with watching the kids in a pinch. In contrast, the neighbour across the street is an extravert. She didn't hesitate to take over some muffins when the new neighbours moved in. The new neighbours were gluten-intolerant and they all had a big laugh about good intentions gone wrong and became fast friends. They watched each other's children after school to give the other parent a break. When a family member became sick suddenly, the neighbour watched their children and took care of the house. Two radically different outcomes, rooted in a decision (or lack thereof) that was ultimately the result of how anxiety-provoking (or not) the idea of meeting a new person would be.

This is how our genotypes influence our environments—by influencing a million tiny little decisions that all impact the way our lives unfold. It starts in infancy and continues throughout our lives, with our genes nudging us in one direction or another, often unbeknownst to ourselves. Researchers call this type of gene–environment correlation *evocative*. We evoke different reactions from the world based on our genetically influenced characteristics. Our temperaments, but also many other pieces of ourselves that are genetically influenced—our appearance, our intelligence, our mental health, our behaviour—all impact our experiences in the world. And to take that a step further, the world around us then responds to our unique genetic code to create a sort of feedback loop. Happy babies are more likely to be smiled at and held. No one wants to hold a stranger's screaming baby. And let's be honest, even parents don't like their own screaming baby after a while!

But there's more—and this brings us to another way that our genotypes and our environments are related. Not only do we evoke certain responses from the world, our genotypes also influence the responses that the world evokes from us. We interpret and react to the world in different ways, based in part on our genetic temperaments. Think back to a recent interaction you may have had at a party. You and a friend end up by the food table locked into a conversation with a stranger who was also reaching for a cheese biscuit. It turns out that she is in the same industry as you and your friend, and she plays the "name game" for a while. You walk away from the conversation and turn to your friend and say, "What a bore and name-dropper; let's stay away from the cheese biscuits". Your friend looks at you in disbelief and says, "I thought she was so friendly! She was trying to make a connection with us". Same interaction, but each person experienced it in a different way.

This kind of difference is called *reactive* gene–environment correlations. Our temperaments influence our reactions to the things we encounter in life. This is why two children growing up in the same family, with the same parents, can actually have very different experiences and memories of their parents. On the one hand, a child with a more sensitive, emotionally reactive temperament may get quite upset when their parent raises their voice at them. They may find the experience frightening, or it may cause them to withdraw from their parent and feel less close to them. On the other hand, another child—even a sibling in the same family—who is less emotionally reactive may be unfazed when their parent raises their voice. It is a non-event for them. Objectively, the parent is doing the same thing with their two children. But the experience of being with that parent is completely different for the two children based on their genetically influenced temperaments. *This also underscores why understanding your child's temperament can help you parent.* The "same" environment is actually not the same, depending on the child's genetic disposition.

Way 2: Active Gene-Environment Correlation

My sister Jeanine and I are two years apart, and as adults we're close. That wasn't always the case. I couldn't stand my sister growing up (sorry, Jeanine, I love you). She was so annoyingly perfect, and it just made me look worse! This really came to a head in secondary school. I was generally a pretty good kid (as I liked to remind my parents repeatedly). But I liked to push the edge of the envelope. If my curfew was midnight, I'd slide in at 12:10 a.m. I snuck out to parties that I wasn't supposed to be at, and sweet-talked my way into bars when I was underage. (But at least I had straight As, right? My parents didn't buy that either.) My sister, meanwhile, spent her weekends at the movies with friends, or hanging out at her friends' houses, under the supervision of parents. Our high school experiences were very different. We attended the same school, we were surrounded by the same environment, but we sought out very different experiences, and those experiences shaped us in different ways. My sister and I have very different temperaments. I was always the more extraverted risk-taker. My sister was more introverted and more anxious. "You're going to get in trouble!" she would say, on the rare occasion that she knew what I was up to as I headed out to an unsanctioned party. Of course, I knew that was a possibility. But the idea of the fun that was to be had led me off to the party anyway, while my sister, for whom the idea of a potential showdown with my parents was far more anxiety-provoking, sensibly chose to head out to a friend's house for a night of movies and popcorn.

This brings us to the second way that our genes influence our environments: *we actively seek out different environments depending on our genetic predispositions.* Sensation-seeking adolescents like to be at parties; the idea of being at a big party probably sounds awful to a more introverted or anxiety-prone adolescent. Some people love the idea of an afternoon wandering around a museum; for others, that sounds like a bore. Some people like going out to eat; others prefer to stay home. Our temperaments shape the environments we seek out and the situations we select ourselves into. This is called *niche-picking*. We pick out our own niches that suit us best. And our genes influence those selections.

As you might expect, active selection of our environments increases as we get older. Children have a limited ability to select their environments. For the most part, your toddler goes where you take him or her. Kids' ability to shape their environments is primarily through their behavioural responses to certain environments. You might try to put your child in theatre classes, but if they hate being onstage and freak out every time you try to drop them off, chances are you'll abandon acting class. If you take your child to a museum and they love looking at the art and you have a fun afternoon together, you're likely to take your child to more museums. Then again, if your child runs wild around the museum and you spend most of the afternoon disciplining him/her and apologising to the museum staff, then you are less likely to seek out more museum bonding experiences in the future. Through their reactions to certain environments, children indirectly shape the experiences that the adults in their life seek out for them. But generally, as a child, you're along for the ride.

Not so as you get older. Adolescents have much more ability to shape their environments than small children do. They can more readily choose their friends (mums and dads are rarely the drivers of "playdates" anymore), and adolescents have more control over how they spend their time. Once they become young adults and leave the home, all bets are off. Now they are the drivers behind where they go and with whom they spend their time. And guess what: those choices are not random. Those choices are shaped by their genetically influenced characteristics (and, we can hope, somewhat by the messaging they have received from influential adults along the way). Adolescents who are more academically oriented hang out at the library and join the chess club. Adolescents who are risk-takers find other fun-loving, risk-taking adolescents. They go skydiving, and join ski racing clubs. They hang out at bars and concerts. Adolescents who are more prone to anxiety or worry spend more time at home in their room. They spend less time engaged in social activities and at parties. Our different genetically influenced temperamental characteristics lead us to seek out different environments and different experiences. And those experiences further shape us.

Way 3: Passive Gene–Environment Correlation

The last way that our genotypes and our environments are intertwined is specific to the parent–child relationship. It is not just our children who have genetically influenced temperaments that affect their environments and their actions. It's true for us adults too. As parents, we also have our own temperamental styles and ways of interacting with the world. These styles influence the way we parent and the environment that we provide for our children. Parents who are more impulsive and risk-taking are more likely to challenge their children to do things that are outside their comfort zone. They are more likely to take them skiing, or skydiving, or sign them up for rock climbing. Parents who are more academic/intellectual types are more likely to create homes filled with books and stacks of *BBC Wildlife* and *the London Review of Books* magazines. Parents who are more introverted may be more likely to plan activities for their children that involve fewer people, and that are quieter in nature. If the idea of being on a stage with everyone looking at you is your idea of hell, then it may not occur to you to sign your child up for theatre classes. Our natural parenting tendencies are in many ways a reflection of our own genetically influenced temperaments.

And here's the kicker: because (biological) parents provide both genes and environments for their kids (remember, kids are a mix-up of 50 per cent mum and 50 per cent dad), it means that children's environments are related to their own genotypes, because those environments are a creation of their parents' genotypes, which the kids also share. In other words, parents' genotypes influence the environments that they provide for their children *and* parents pass their genetic material on to their children. This means that even for small children, their environments (assuming they were provided by a biological parent) are correlated with their genotypes.

Let's imagine, for example, a parent with a high IQ. We know that intelligence is heritable, meaning that our genes play a role in cognitive ability. A parent with a high IQ is more likely to pass along high-IQ genes to their kids, and also more likely to create a house full of books. That means that their children are more likely to have an edge when it comes to their genetic predispositions *and* to have the advantage of having lots of books to further stimulate their academic disposition. Their parents may be more likely to send them to academically enriching summer activity camps because those are the things they enjoyed. So their already advantaged kids get another "environmental" boost from Lego Squad and summer engineering. Their intelligent parents are more likely to be able to help with homework and to be excited when their children show a shared love of learning. These kids are essentially getting a double whammy of enriched genes *and* an enhanced environment, stemming from their parents' above-average intelligence, which is where it all started.

The flip side is unfortunately true too—kids can get a double dose of disadvantaged effects. For example, we know that aggression is significantly genetically influenced. This means that children who inherit an aggressive temperament are also more likely to have aggressive parents. This can create a home environment characterised by harsh parenting or punitive punishment. These environmental experiences may serve to further exacerbate the child's tendency towards aggression. These children got an unfortunate roll of the genetic dice in terms of being more quick to temper, and then they have an environment that models and further stokes that behaviour.

You've probably already realised that passive gene–environment correlation exists only when kids are raised by biological relatives. Children who are adopted into families and parented by non-relatives do not necessarily have environments that are related to their genotypes. Evocative/reactive gene–environment correlation and active gene–environment correlation still play a role, however, no matter who raises the children. Even without home environments related to their genotypes, all children's genotypes influence the responses they evoke from the individuals in their lives, how they react to their environments, and the environments that they seek out in the first place.

The Role of Cascading Developmental Effects

So, let's return to the studies of identical twins reared apart that we discussed in chapter 1. As you read about this research, you may have wondered: how is it possible that identical twins who grow up in different environments can be just as similar as identical twins who grow up together? Let's revisit these findings through the lens of what you now know about gene–environment correlation. The twins were raised by different sets of adoptive parents, so their home environments were not by default correlated with their genotypes (no passive gene–environment interaction). But they shared the same genetic code, so they started life with similar temperaments. Those temperaments were likely to evoke similar responses—from their (different) parents, from their teachers, and more generally from the people they encountered in the world. They were raised separately, so they had their own lives; but because their environmental experiences, and their reactions to them, were influenced by their genetically influenced characteristics, they were having more similar experiences than two random people would as they moved through their lives. And over time, similar feedback from the world, and interpretations of life events, increasingly shaped them to be similar people. In other words, a big part of our "environmental experiences" actually start with our genes. That's likely how the famous Jim twins turned out to be so similar, despite being raised by different parents.

Of course, some environmental events really are random. Experiencing a natural disaster, such as an earthquake or a hurricane, is not likely to be related to your genes. Other kinds of stressful events, like car accidents, may or may not be related to your genetic make-up. Some car accidents are random: you were in the wrong place at the wrong time, and a distracted driver ran a red light and hit you. But maybe the car accident happened in part because you were speeding (because you're a risk-taker!) or because you weren't fully focused, because you've been struggling with depression and couldn't concentrate. Sometimes even seemingly "random" environmental events are partially influenced by our own characteristics. In Japan, they take this to the extreme when assigning fault in car accidents. Both parties are always partially at fault, if only by being present when someone hit them!

Aside from the "slings and arrows of outrageous fortune", our genes impact a number of aspects of our environment. And even when we experience random events, both good and bad, our genes influence the way we react to them. It's the feedback loop of life, set in motion by each child's unique genetic make-up.

The Role of a Good Parent:
Fine-Tuning Your Child's Disposition

So where do parents come in? Our children's genes lay the foundation for their dispositions, and they influence the way our children move through the world, but their genes *do not* write their destiny. By working with your child's genetic disposition, you can nudge them towards their best possible self, and help them to control their natural tendencies that may lead them into trouble. In other words, environments can influence how genetic predispositions are expressed. We call this *gene–environment interaction*.

For parents this means, for example, that if you have a child naturally disposed to impulsivity, you can set boundaries to help them learn to control their impulsive nature, and by doing so, you can help curb those impulsive tendencies and the likelihood that those tendencies will get them into trouble. If you have a child disposed to high emotionality (or what we as parents tend to call "freaking out over nothing"), you can help your child learn to manage their emotionality, and by doing so, help keep their genetic disposition in check. You can also help nurture your child's natural genetic strengths so that they blossom further. For example, a child who naturally loves being around others will thrive in an environment where they interact with more children, which can further contribute to developing social skills.

By understanding your child's disposition, you can have a better idea of what environments will help them succeed, and which ones they may be drawn to that will get them into trouble. Gene–environment interaction means that as parents we can help tune up or tune down certain genetic tendencies, like the volume knob on a radio. Unfortunately, we're usually not in charge of the on/off button (though I have admittedly fantasised about it when my child was throwing a fit). But the science suggests that the tuning process is one of the ways parents can have their biggest impact.

Back in the 1960s, my first mentor, Irving Gottesman, a clinical psychologist and founding father in the field of behaviour genetics, introduced the idea of *reaction range* as a way of thinking about how genes and environment work together to shape how children turn out. *Reaction range* refers to the idea that we may start life with a certain genetic disposition, but the environment will shape how that disposition unfolds. For example, you can imagine a child who is naturally disposed towards introversion and prefers time alone. As a parent, you can help that child learn to be more comfortable around others by gently and persistently exposing them to other children, rather than allowing them to stay solo in their room all the time. Doing this will help them grow up to be comfortable in a social setting when needed, even if it is not their preferred activity. But regardless of what you do, you're probably not going to be able to parent that naturally introverted child to want to stand out as the life of the party, like a more extraverted child might.

Conversely, if you have a highly extraverted child, you might want to focus your parenting on helping your child channel their disposition into social outlets like starring in the school play or public speaking, so that they are *less* likely to end up dancing on tables in bars! In other words, genetic dispositions set boundaries within which our kids develop, but their environments will interact with their genetic dispositions to influence where they end up. As parents we can think of our job as trying to bring out our child's best dispositions, and help them manage their less advantageous tendencies (because we all have those too).

There's one last genetic concept that's important to understand: epigenetics. Epigenetics is related to gene–environment interaction. It refers to the fact that environments can influence the expression of genes at the molecular level. Environmental experiences can influence whether genes get turned on or off, or the degree to which they get expressed. New research suggests that stressful environments can have adverse epigenetic effects, activating genes involved in stress response, and leading to a cascade of adverse physical, behavioural, and psychological outcomes. Neighbourhoods where poverty or crime are prevalent, childhood trauma, discrimination—all of these factors have been shown to alter gene expression and adversely affect child development in ways that can be transmitted across generations. Super-parenting our kids won't shape them in the way we might have imagined, but stressful and traumatic experiences *can* hurt our children and impede their ability to reach their potential.

Now that you have a basic understanding of the ways that genes and environments work together to impact children's behaviour, Part 2 of *The Child Code* will help you identify *your child's* unique genetic tendencies and learn how to parent their distinct mix of genes. This knowledge will enable you to influence the pathways through which their genes and environments intermingle across time to shape their development.

Takeaways

- There are no genes "for" behaviour. Our genes shape our lives in more complicated and indirect ways.

- Complex behaviours are influenced by many genes—probably hundreds or thousands—that all come together to impact our natural tendency towards that behaviour, whether it is impulsivity, anxiety, extraversion, or any other behavioural tendency. Genes shape our behaviour by influencing how our brains are wired.

- Our genetically influenced characteristics, from our temperament to our appearance, influence our experience in the world. Children with different genetic tendencies evoke different reactions from the people around them, which further shapes their development.

- We interpret and react to the world in different ways, based on our genetic temperament. This is why two children growing up in the same family, with the same parents, can actually have very different experiences with their parents, because they have unique genetic dispositions.

- Our genotypes influence the environments we seek out. For example, highly extraverted children seek out active environments with lots of people.

- Children respond to their parents and their home environments in different ways based on their genetically influenced temperament. This is why what works for one child is just as likely to not work for another child.

- By working with your child's genetic disposition, you can help them navigate their world. Parents can tune up or tune down children's dispositions; the environment can change the expression of children's genotypes.

PART 2

Building Blocks

. . . ▬ . . .

CHAPTER 3

Getting to Know Your Child: "The Big Three" Dimensions of Temperament

Years ago, my best friend from college and I were in a playground with our small children, who were playing on the climbing frame. My son had climbed up and was standing spread-eagle at the top shouting, "Look at me!" Her son was looking at him dubiously from the ground, and timidly offered, "I don't think that's a good idea . . ." To which my child yelled back, "But it's so much fun!"

We learn about our children's natural dispositions by observing their behaviour. As parents, part of our job is to be a loving detective. That comes naturally when our children are infants. When our babies cry we have to figure out whether they need feeding, a nappy change, a nap, or a blanket, and then we act accordingly. Before too long, we figure out the "I'm hungry!" cry versus the "I'm tired!" cry.

As a parent, you know your child better than anyone, and you use this knowledge to attend to their basic needs when they are infants. *But it doesn't stop there.* Learning your child's tendencies—tendencies that will differ for each child—can help you adapt your parenting to give your child what they need across all stages of development. It can also help you avoid the frustration of failing with ineffective, off-the-record parenting techniques that are never going to work with your kid. Part of your detective role is figuring out what works—and what doesn't—for your unique bundle of genes.

My friend's child was naturally more fearful and timid, so as a parent, she had to focus on encouraging him to try new things, to get him out of his comfort zone, and to take a bit more risk. That's the last thing my child needed! My child's tendencies towards fearlessness and impulsivity meant that I had to focus on teaching him self-control, and helping him avoid situations that could put him in danger. She had to adopt a soft, persistent, patient parenting style. My child needed firmer boundaries. Gentle redirection didn't work well with my son, just as firm, directive parenting would have been harder on her more sensitive child. Admittedly, it took some detective work to figure this out. My natural tendency is to talk things through (there's a reason I chose to be a psychologist!). But after repeated conversations resulted in no change to my son's impulsive behaviour, I discovered that simple, firm rules did a much better job.

Imagine two children, we'll call them Alexis and Caleb, who both start out as fearful toddlers. Their genetic make-up has coded for brains that naturally predispose them towards more anxiety. Alexis and Caleb cling to their respective mother's legs when strangers stop to talk. They hang back and don't want to play with the other children at the playground. They sit at the edge of the pool and cry when their parents try to enroll them in swimming lessons. But Alexis and Caleb's respective parents take very different approaches to managing their naturally more fearful temperaments.

As Caleb hides behind their legs, his parents explain to friends that he's very shy and resume their conversation, not wanting to embarrass him. They play with him one-on-one on the playground rather than try to persuade him to interact with other children. When Caleb refuses to get into the pool at swimming lessons, his parents explain to the teacher that he must not be ready yet and take him home to try again next year.

Conversely, when Alexis hides in the presence of new individuals, her parents gently coax her out and patiently wait for her to come say hello before resuming their conversation with friends. When she is afraid to approach the other children in the playground, they take her over and introduce her and stay with her near the other children until she gets comfortable. When Alexis refuses to get into the pool, they continue to bring her to every class and have her sit beside the pool until she's ready to get in.

What's important to realise here is that neither Alexis nor Caleb's parents are doing anything "wrong." They both have their child's best interests at heart and are responding to their children and adapting their parenting as best they can. But the strategy that Alexis's parents take—gently, slowly, patiently introducing and exposing their fearful child to situations they would naturally avoid—is a far more effective way to help children (and adults!) slowly conquer fear.

Caleb's parents, although equally well-meaning, aren't helping their son in the long run. By adapting in a way that protects him from his fears, they never help him learn to master his natural inclination towards anxiety.

The Three Es

Researchers have lots of ways of slicing and dicing temperament. There are dozens of measures of temperament, and different experts have different ways of categorising and naming dimensions of temperament and behaviour. In *The Child Code*, I'm going to focus on three big traits that have consistently emerged (though with slightly different names and nuances) across hundreds of studies examining behavioural tendencies in infants and young children. These studies have used reports from parents and other important individuals in children's lives, as well as observations of children's behaviour in research laboratories and in natural settings like the home. The "Three Es," or the "Big Three" (as I like to call them), show up across children from different cultures, and across genders (with some small gender differences, which we'll discuss later). They tap dimensions that can first be detected in infants, and that show consistency into early and middle childhood.

The Three Es isn't a phrase you will come across in the scholarly literature. This is me as a parent, extracting lots of information from vast and complicated scientific literatures, to create a tool kit of useful information for parents. So, for the researcher–parents out there, know that this book is not intended to be a review of the literature. It's a parent's translation of findings from clinical psychology, developmental psychology, and behaviour genetics (the fields across which I am trained), put together in a way intended to maximise its utility for other parents.

The Big Three dimensions give you a window into your child's underlying genetic make-up. They predict behaviour in adolescence, and into adulthood. Closely observing and understanding where your child falls on these dimensions is a big part of your job as a parent. Finding a parenting approach that will work for you begins with knowing who your child is, in terms of genetic design.

I'm going to introduce you to six children who represent the high and low end of each of the Big Three dimensions. As you're reading about these children with different temperamental traits, it's critical to remember that there are no inherently "good" or "bad" traits. Yes, children with certain predispositions can be more challenging for parents. But whether we view characteristics as "good" or "bad" can actually change across time, and across cultures. As we discussed earlier in the book, some of the things that seem good with young kids (for example, sociability) actually make for difficult teenagers (more sociable teenagers are more likely to be influenced by peers and experiment with alcohol and other drugs). Some of the traits that are challenging in children (refusal to comply) are valued in adults (standing up for your principles). Some cultures place greater importance on obedience in children, whereas others emphasise individuality. The point is, dispositions all come with pluses and minuses (though admittedly some of them make parenting more challenging at various developmental stages).

Extraversion: Lila and Mila

Lila's parents joked that she came out ready to take the world by storm. As a baby, she loved to play peek-a-boo, and would belly-laugh over and over as her parents played with her. She delighted at new toys. She seemed to love going on outings with her parents. As a baby, she cooed at strangers who stopped to peek into her pram as she and her parents went for a walk in the neighbourhood. Once Lila started crawling, she was always on the go. She loved Little Gym classes, and the parent–child sing-along music sessions. She eagerly explored new playgrounds and easily made friends with other children she met at the park. She loved shopping, and ran excitedly through the supermarket "helpfully" placing items in the trolley. Her parents had a rule of thumb that if they didn't take Lila outside to burn off some energy, something inevitably got broken as Lila cheerfully ran around, "flying" her airplanes through the house or jumping into the pillow fort she had built in the study.

Mila, by contrast, was a quiet, contented baby. She was happy to lie in her parents' arms, looking up at them peacefully. She infrequently squirmed or tried to wiggle away from them. High-intensity games like peek-a-boo seemed to be too much for her; she preferred just to snuggle. She would sit quietly as books were read to her. As she got older, she preferred to stay at the house and play quiet games, like the card game Memory, rather than to go to a noisy playground or to the mall play area. She was shy at first when new people came to the house, and it took her a little while to warm up to strangers. But after a short period, she would happily show them her stuffed animals and "host" a small tea party in her room. When the house got quiet, Mila's parents knew they would usually find her in her room playing with blocks or doing a puzzle.

Lila and Mila represent children who fall on opposite ends of the first dimension of the Big Three Es: *Extraversion*. The roots of Extraversion show up early in development, and they're reflected in a child's natural tendencies towards positive affect (how delighted they are by the world and other people); activity level (how much children are "on the move"); and exploratory behaviour (how much children like trying new things).

Children who are high on Extraversion tend to be happy and active. As babies, they laugh easily and often. They make cooing sounds when their parents engage with them. They tend to be more on the go, squirming around in mum or dad's arms, moving around on their play mats. Highly extraverted children enjoy going to new places. They find new activities exciting. As they grow older, they are full of energy—they prefer playing at the playground or going down high slides. They run rather than walk from one place to another. They enjoy meeting new people.

At the other end of this dimension are children who are naturally quieter and less active. As babies, they are content to lie in your arms quietly. Children who are lower on Extraversion are shyer with strangers, and sometimes even with people they have met before but don't see regularly. They are more content to play by themselves, or with a small group. They don't need to be surrounded by a bustle of activity or people, and often would prefer not to be.

Emotionality: Chloe and Zoe

From the time she was born, Chloe didn't like being set down or held by strangers. She would get very upset when her parents tried to put her in the bouncy chair, crying intensely until her parents picked her back up again. They tried a host of baby products that their friends swore by, but Chloe didn't seem to like any of them. When she was upset, it was difficult to settle her down. When she was tired, everything seemed to get even more challenging. She was very reactive to anything that she didn't like. Sometimes her parents couldn't even figure out what she was upset about. She resisted going to bed or going down for her nap, even though her parents could tell she was tired. As she got older, she continued to get very upset when things didn't go her way. If she lost at a game, or her art project didn't turn out as she had hoped, she would throw huge fits, and her parents had trouble consoling her or redirecting the behaviour. She could be fearful of strangers. When her mum signed her up for a playgroup, she refused to go inside and threw herself on the ground screaming and kicking when her parent tried to get her to participate.

By contrast, Zoe is what her parents would describe as "go with the flow". She soothed easily as a baby. She allowed multiple adults to hold her, and she would contentedly sit in her swing or lie on her activity mat. When she was a toddler, her parents could redirect her when she got upset. Though there might be tears because her favourite cereal was gone, she quickly rebounded and was content again when her parents suggested they could play a game after she finished breakfast. She's generally happy doing whatever activities her parents have planned for her, whether it's an outing to a children's museum or a day of craft projects. Although she might be hesitant to go to a playground where she doesn't know the other children, she doesn't get overly distressed and will slowly join in with the other children.

Chloe and Zoe represent children who fall on opposite ends of the Big Three dimension of *Emotionality*. Children who are high on Emotionality are naturally more prone to distress, fear, and frustration. As babies and small children, they are more likely to get upset, especially when they are tired. They'll cry when a toy is removed from them, and resist going to bed or going down for naps, even though they are tired. As small children, they may get very distressed if they can't do something that they set out to do, whether that is winning a favourite game or playing a sport. Their upset can be perceived as "overreacting". They not only get easily frustrated or angry, but they stay that way for what feels like a long time. Children who are high on Emotionality don't redirect easily. They are more likely to be fearful, afraid of monsters at night or someone breaking into the house. It was on the fear subdimension of Emotionality that Caleb and Alexis, the children described earlier in this chapter, differed so radically.

Effortful Control: Hayden and Jayden

Hayden is a child who can sit quietly while his parents read to him. When he starts building a castle with blocks, he will focus for hours. When doing a puzzle, he can concentrate for long periods of time until the task is done. He is good at following his parents' directions. If he has to complete a task before getting a treat, or wait until after dinner for an ice lolly, he can do so without getting very upset. When he is at the playground and his parents call to him, he comes right over. When they ask him to stop doing something, he stops.

Jayden, by contrast, flits from one activity to another. He starts a puzzle, but quickly becomes bored and starts another activity. His parents will often find a number of projects underway in his room, in varying stages of completion. He has trouble sitting through activities if they take more than ten minutes or so. He doesn't like to sit still for more than one book. When engaged in a playful sword fight with his younger brother, he gets carried away. Often when his parents ask him to stop doing something, it takes multiple requests before he complies. When asked to wait for a treat, he has a lot of trouble. If Jayden knows where the biscuits are, he'll be caught with the proverbial hand in the biscuit jar!

Hayden and Jayden differ on the final dimension of the Big Three: *Effortful Control*. In children, Effortful Control is often referred to as *self-control*. After the first year of life, children start developing the ability to regulate their emotions and behaviour. Early on, Effortful Control shows up in how well children regulate their emotions and can focus their attention. As they get older, Effortful Control shows up in whether small children can focus on playing with a single toy, and in how well they can follow instructions, or hold back from doing things they aren't supposed to do.

Figuring Out Your Child

As you've been reading the descriptions of the children in this chapter, you've probably been thinking about how your child compares. Are they more of a Lila or a Mila? A Chloe or a Zoe? A Hayden or a Jayden? For some dimensions it may be obvious. But for others, it may take more time and observation to figure out your child, in your loving detective role. As you try to evaluate where your child lies on the Big Three continuum, there are some things you should keep in mind:

Look for consistency across situations. All children are sometimes fearful, sometimes happy, sometimes grumpy, sometimes aggressive, so when we talk about genetically influenced temperaments, we're talking about tendencies that show *consistency across situations*. That's why in describing the different children above, I mentioned a variety of different ways that the tendency manifests. In deciding where your child falls, you want to think about how often *the range of behaviours* applies and not just whether they ever display one of the relevant behaviours. Most children will display fear if a dog suddenly starts snarling, growling, and lunging at them (most adults would too!). But a fearful child is one who is scared of dogs even when they're politely going about their doggie business. And it's not just about fear of dogs. It's about being consistently fearful of being away from the parent, of meeting new people, of going new places—you name it.

Think about consistency across time. Genetically influenced traits also show *consistency across time*. That means that you will have a better idea of your child's innate genetic tendencies as they grow. Many temperamental characteristics start showing up as early as two to three months, but the more time you spend with your child, the more you will start to identify what is a truly stable characteristic versus just a developmental phase. For example, it's normal for toddlers to go through a phase of exerting their independence and displaying the charming behaviour of responding to all your requests with an adamant "No!" This

61

does not necessarily mean that you have a child who is destined to grow into a defiant teenager—it just means you have a toddler. Temperament really starts to solidify by age three, so the older your child is, the more accurately you can assess their genetic disposition. Genes influence the extent to which a behaviour is stable across time, so behaviours that your child consistently displays as they get older are more accurate reflections of their genetic dispositions. If your fearful toddler who cowers at the petting zoo and refuses to go to Little Gym subsequently goes on to be afraid to start kindergarten and baulks at the idea of playdates with friends, over time you can feel more confident that this is not a phase, but a disposition towards anxiety in your child.

Consider your child's age. Keep in mind that because underlying differences are a reflection of the different ways that our brains are wired, and children have rapidly developing brains, different traits show up at different points in child development. Behaviours related to Extra-version and Emotionality show up early. Infants differ in how much they smile and laugh (Extraversion: Positive Affect), and how much they show distress and frustration (Emotionality). They differ in how much they move around (Extraversion: Activity), and whether they like exploring new places or toys (Extraversion: Exploration). Fear of new things starts to show up towards the end of the first year of life (Emotionality). And Effortful Control (unfortunately for us parents) shows up last, emerging after the first year of life, then developing rapidly between ages two and seven. The point to remember is that depending on how old your child is, you may not yet have had a chance to observe all their natural tenden-cies in all these areas.

Consider your own bias. Just as our children experience the world based on their natural tendencies, our own genetic predispositions also influence how *we* see the world as parents, which influences the way we interpret our children's behaviour. A parent whose natural tendency is to be more cautious may view their child's rambunctious behaviour as far more impulsive than would a parent who is naturally more of a thrill-seeker themselves. As you try to gauge your child's innate tendencies, it can be helpful to have other trusted adults in the child's life—for example, your partner or a caregiver or grandparent who spend a lot of time with the child—also indicate where they see the child falling on each temperamental dimension.

Last but not least: Be honest. As you're mapping out your child's natural tendencies, this is no time to be worried about what your mother thinks or how you imagine your child *should* be. You're trying to understand their genetically influenced tendencies so that you can figure out how best to parent them and to increase harmony in your home. Some dispositions may initially seem more desirable than others, but again, dispositions are not inherently good or bad. Nor are they destiny. You have to be true to your child, because that's the only way to know how to be the best parent for them.

Your Child and the Three Es

At the end of this chapter is the "All About Your Child" survey, which consists of a series of questions that tap into each of the Big Three dimensions to help you figure out your child's natural dispositions. Remember that the older your child is, the more accurately you can assess where he or she falls across the Big Three Es. The next several chapters will walk you through each of the Big Three dimensions, and combinations thereof, and dive more deeply into what it means for your child if they are high/medium/low on Extraversion, high/medium/low on Emotionality, and high/medium/low on Effortful Control. You'll note that I am very intentional throughout this book about describing children as falling *across a continuum* on the Three Es; I use high/medium/low as shorthand, but in general I do not use labels (with the exception of extravert/introvert in chapter 4, since that is such common vernacular for high and low Extraversion).

A lot of personality tests do assign labels. This practice dates all the way back to the ancient Greeks, who relegated people to four personality types: sanguine, choleric, melancholic, and phlegmatic (ewww). The Myers-Briggs Type Indicator famously assigns people to four categories (introversion or extraversion; sensing or intuition; thinking or feeling; and judging or perceiving), with four-letter "types" produced (shout out to my fellow ESTJs). Even Harry Potter and the Hogwarts students got sorted into houses.

It can be fun to identify with a group, and there are even evolutionary reasons why people may be drawn to groups; there can be safety and affinity associated with being part of a group. But when it comes to personality and temperament, humans vary *continuously*, rather than falling into distinct classes. In other words, our genes impact *how much* of that characteristic comes to us naturally. The way those predispositions play out will vary as a function of our environments. For example, you can teach a child who is naturally low on Effortful Control skills to help them build their self-control (we'll get into that in chapter 6). That isn't guaranteed to convert them to a highly regulated child who wants to sit quietly for hours, but it can at least cut down on the number of times you catch them up to mischief. Remembering that behaviour is on a continuum can remind us that change is possible.

In the chapters that follow, we will discuss the strengths associated with different dispositions, and the challenges that can come with each dispositional style (for both children and their parents!). We'll talk about what types of parenting strategies are most effective for different children. In short, the next few chapters will help you put what you've learned to work, giving you a road map to *help you* guide your one-of-a-kind offspring, and to help you *help them* navigate the world. In child development, we call this *Goodness of Fit*.

Goodness of Fit

Goodness of Fit refers to the match between children and their parents, as well as the child's environment more broadly. Goodness of Fit is critical to having a happy, stress-free (or at least lower-stress!) home life. Some parents and children are lucky enough to have a natural Goodness of Fit. Mum is a bookworm, for example, and her daughter loves being read to. Mum takes her daughter to toddler reading time at the local library, and they spend quality time together afterwards, picking out books and snuggling up together in the reading nook. They also share a love of doing puzzles or colouring side by side. Or maybe Mum was a star athlete. She loves sports and being at sporting events. She signs her daughter up for sports lessons as early as she can, and they do family outings to local rugby and football events, which her child loves. They enjoy cheering together with other fans at the matches.

When there is natural Goodness of Fit with their environment, children thrive, and parents generally don't recognise the underlying reason. Parenting their child simply feels "easy". In this scenario, parents often attribute their child's love of books or sports to the parents' exposing the child to that environment. And certainly, some of that is true. But remember from chapter 1 that parent–child similarity doesn't actually mean that the parent is influencing the child's behaviour. What parents often fail to appreciate is that often it is just a lucky match. In the first example above, mum and daughter are both low on Extraversion and high on Effortful Control. Quiet activities like reading at a library or doing puzzles together appeal to both of them. In the second example, mum and daughter are both high on Extraversion. They like being around people and on the go. Active, busy events like sports are appealing to them. It turns out athletic ability is actually genetically influenced too, so they may also be matched on that front as well.

But imagine what happens when bookworm mum, who prefers quiet time at the library, has a child who is high on Extraversion and low on Effortful Control. Mum's repeated attempts to read to her daughter are unsuccessful, as her daughter shows no interest in sitting still and looking at the book, instead jumping off mum's lap to gallop her hobby horse around the room. During toddler time at the library, much to her mother's embarrassment, her daughter repeatedly gets up and wants to run around the library, pulling a book off the shelf, then sprinting on to the next one after a quick glance at the cover. As this happens week after week, mum gets increasingly frustrated with her daughter and feels like she is constantly having to discipline her child rather than enjoying their time together.

In the second example, imagine if sporty mum has a child who is low on Extraversion. Mum wants to take her daughter to the Jumping Beans class at the gym, and maybe cheer together at older sister's football match. But her daughter finds all the people and activity to be overwhelming. She constantly pleads with her mum not to go. When mum insists, she sulks in the corner and refuses to participate.

In both cases, mums were well-meaning, trying to give their daughters opportunities that they imagined their children would enjoy while also bonding with their child. But if we're honest, we can see that we tend to provide our children with the things *we* would want, naturally assuming that they will like the things that we like. It's a natural default to assume that other people's brains are wired the way ours are, especially the brains of our children. After all, we only know the lens through which we see the world.

When there is a natural Goodness of Fit between parent and child temperaments, everything works smoothly. But when parents and children have different natural dispositions, especially when parents aren't consciously aware of what's going on, it can lead to increased parent–child friction and a lot of frustration for all concerned. It also can be very damaging for family relations. In both of our example "mismatched" families, the mothers couldn't understand why their daughters were behaving inappropriately, and they found themselves in negative, conflictual cycles. No one wants to spend toddler time at the library constantly telling their child to sit down and behave while the other parents repeatedly send irritated glances her way. No one wants to spend toddler gym time huddled in the corner trying to coax their child to participate while the child is crying and clinging to the door.

What neither of these mothers understood was that the respective activities they were planning for their children simply weren't a good fit for their child's temperament. When children who are mismatched with their activities are also high on Emotionality, the result can be temper tantrums and staunch refusal to participate.

Understanding Goodness of Fit doesn't mean that you are a slave to your child's dispositions, but it will equip you to make better decisions and to anticipate which kinds of activities are likely to be a natural fit and what kinds are likely to require a thoughtful strategy.

Understanding Your Profile

There's one last piece to providing Goodness of Fit. As you may have realised from the above examples, Goodness of Fit isn't just about your child's natural dispositions, it's also about *yours*. As we discussed, we all have different genetically influenced dispositions, and they affect the way we parent and respond to our children. For example, one parent may find it incredibly anxiety-provoking to have a child who is high on Extraversion and low on Effortful Control, prompting constant fears of having to rush to the ER. That same behaviour in a child who has a parent with a different temperament might elicit a proud pat on the back accompanied by "Wow! Look at you!" For that reason, providing a Goodness of Fit for your child requires you to be mindful in assessing yourself, as well as your child.

Following the "All About Your Child" survey, you'll find a survey that is "All About You". This survey will give you a window into your own natural tendencies, which reflect your genetic predispositions, combined with years of lived experience.

The surveys are tools to help you evaluate where you and your child fall on each of the Big Three dimensions, along with a summary sheet to compare your dispositions. This information will serve as the foundation for the following chapters, which will dive in to help you better understand your child, how your child evokes certain responses in you, and how to create a Goodness of Fit with your child. Ultimately, understanding the dynamic interplay between you and your child will allow you to have a happier, more enjoyable coexistence and help you to unlock your child's potential.

Adopting the Right Mindset

There's one last piece to consider before you jump into the surveys. Understanding your child's natural dispositions can help you as a parent, but you want to be careful not to fall into a fixed mindset, believing your child's tendencies are set in stone ("My child is high on Emotionality, so they will never change and I'm doomed to a lifetime of fits"). *Nothing about the way genes work indicates this is true.* Yes, predispositions influence our children's behaviour in profound ways, and this can allow us to anticipate challenges and help our children work through them. It can also help us recognise and build on their natural strengths. Understanding our children can help *us* help *them* to grow.

Psychologist Carol Dweck has written extensively about the power of a *growth mindset*, as compared to a *fixed mindset*. A growth mindset involves believing you can cultivate your natural abilities through effort, applying strategies, and with help from others. That is exactly what the next several chapters will help you do—recognise your child's natural tendencies and how you can adopt strategies to help them reach their full potential. Dweck's research has shown that the way you see yourself can have a profound influence on the way your life unfolds. By extension, the way we see our children can have a profound influence on the way *their* lives unfold.

Dweck points out that, as parents, our hopes and dreams for our children can easily translate into a fixed mindset, meaning that we cling to the mould we want our child to fit, whether that is a brilliant student, talented artist, star of the school play, Oxbridge graduate—or, I might add, just a well-behaved child who wants to spend afternoons at the library or enjoying sports together. When our children's natural proclivities don't match our ideas, we may inadvertently send the message to our children that we are judging them for who they are (or who they are not). Further, when our children have setbacks—which they inevitably will—and as parents we jump to worrying about what that means for their future, it reflects a fixed mindset. If they don't have the self-control to sit quietly and focus now, how will they ever graduate from university, or get a job?! It conveys to our children that we don't have confidence in their ability to grow, change, and realise their potential.

The surveys that follow will help you understand your child's natural tendencies, but keep in mind that human development is a *process*. One of the greatest roles you can play as a parent is to help your child recognise and appreciate their own unique talents and penchants, overcome their challenges, and grow into their best possible selves.

The "All About Your Child" Survey

Listed below are a set of descriptions of ways children can respond to a variety of situations. For each question, try to think about how your child *typically* reacts. Depending on the age of your child, some items will be more appropriate than others. For each statement, make a mark on the line below, indicating the extent to which the statement is completely *untrue* of your child (far left) to completely *true* of your child (far right). If the statement seems neither fully true nor false about your child, put a mark in the middle. Try to use the full range of the bar, indicating the extent to which the statement is completely untrue, a little bit untrue, neither fully true or false, a little bit true, or completely true.

EXTRAVERSION (THE "EX" FACTOR)

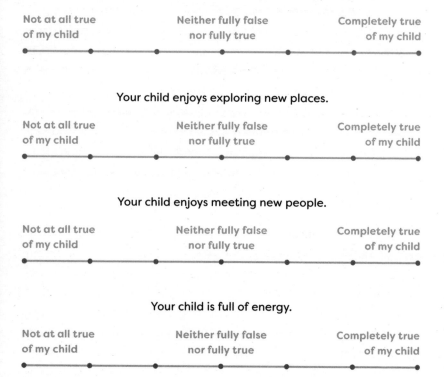

Your child likes adventuresome games or activities.

Not at all true
of my child

Neither fully false
nor fully true

Completely true
of my child

Your child enjoys exploring new places.

Not at all true
of my child

Neither fully false
nor fully true

Completely true
of my child

Your child enjoys meeting new people.

Not at all true
of my child

Neither fully false
nor fully true

Completely true
of my child

Your child is full of energy.

Not at all true
of my child

Neither fully false
nor fully true

Completely true
of my child

Look at where your marks fall on the above questions. If you have a lot of marks on the right side of the bars, your child is naturally predisposed to be high on Extraversion. If most of your marks are on the left side of the bars, then your child is low on Extraversion. Some children fall in the middle of this dimension and are not strongly extraverted or introverted. The following are additional indicators of low Extraversion:

Your child prefers quiet activities, like reading,
over more high energy activities, like running around.

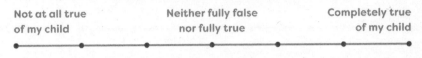

Not at all true
of my child

Neither fully false
nor fully true

Completely true
of my child

Your child takes a long time to warm up to a new person,
or is slow to approach a new situation.

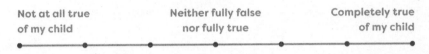

Not at all true
of my child

Neither fully false
nor fully true

Completely true
of my child

Look back at your answers to the above questions about high Extraversion, and the additional indicators of low Extraversion. Where do most of your marks fall? Overall, where does your child fall on Extraversion?

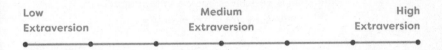

Low
Extraversion

Medium
Extraversion

High
Extraversion

EMOTIONALITY (THE "EM" FACTOR)

Your child gets very frustrated when things don't go their way.

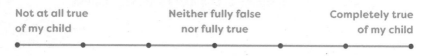

Your child is afraid of monsters or sounds in the night.

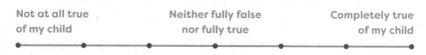

**When your child gets upset, they stay upset
for what seems like a long time, ten minutes or more.**

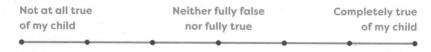

**Your child is difficult to soothe or to redirect
when they are upset or angry.**

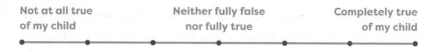

Look at where your marks fall on the above questions. If you have a lot of marks on the right side of the bars, your child is naturally predisposed to be high on Emotionality. If most of your marks are on the left side of the bars, then your child is low on Emotionality. The following are additional indicators of low Emotionality:

**My child does not get overly upset when things don't go as planned.
They are fairly "go with the flow".**

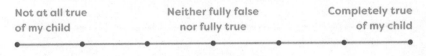

Not at all true
of my child

Neither fully false
nor fully true

Completely true
of my child

**When my child gets upset, they are able to recover
fairly quickly and redirect to a new activity.**

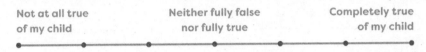

Not at all true
of my child

Neither fully false
nor fully true

Completely true
of my child

Look back at your answers to the above questions about high Emotionality, and the additional indicators of low Emotionality. Where do most of your marks fall? Overall, where does your child fall on Emotionality?

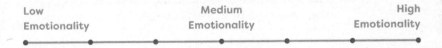

Low
Emotionality

Medium
Emotionality

High
Emotionality

EFFORTFUL CONTROL (THE "EF" FACTOR)

My child can stop a behaviour when told "no".

Not at all true
of my child

Neither fully false
nor fully true

Completely true
of my child

My child shows strong concentration when they are engaged in a single activity, such as colouring or building with blocks.

Not at all true
of my child

Neither fully false
nor fully true

Completely true
of my child

My child is good at following directions.

Not at all true
of my child

Neither fully false
nor fully true

Completely true
of my child

My child is careful when approaching a situation that they have been told is dangerous.

Not at all true
of my child

Neither fully false
nor fully true

Completely true
of my child

My child can wait for a reward when instructed to do so.

Not at all true
of my child

Neither fully false
nor fully true

Completely true
of my child

Look at where your marks fall on the preceding questions. If you have a lot of marks on the right side of the bars, your child is naturally predisposed to be high on Effortful Control. If most of your marks are on the left side of the bars, then your child is low on Effortful Control. The following are additional indicators of low Effortful Control:

My child has trouble waiting their turn or sitting still.

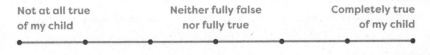

Not at all true	Neither fully false	Completely true
of my child	nor fully true	of my child

My child rushes into activities or situations without thinking them through.

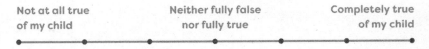

Not at all true	Neither fully false	Completely true
of my child	nor fully true	of my child

Look back at your answers to the earlier questions about high Effortful Control, and the additional indicators of low Effortful Control. Where do most of your marks fall? Overall, where does your child fall on Effortful Control?

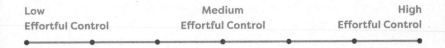

Low	Medium	High
Effortful Control	Effortful Control	Effortful Control

My Child's Profile

Based on your earlier responses, indicate below whether your child is Low, Medium, or High on each of the Big Three Es:

Extraversion (Ex)	Low/Medium/High
Emotionality (Em)	Low/Medium/High
Effortful Control (Ef)	Low/Medium/High

To help you remember your child's disposition, I've provided abbreviations for each dimension: Ex, Em, Ef. For example, you can think about your child as High Ex, High Em, Low Ef (modified to their particular profile). This shorthand (Ex, Em, Ef) provides a quick reference for you to remember your child's temperament.

The "All About You" Survey

Consider the following questions as you think about your own natural dispositions. The questions differ from the child assessment since adults have more developed personalities, influenced by years of lived experience, combined with genetic predispositions. In the following survey, I have roughly mapped different personality styles in adults to related dimensions in children. The purpose of this exercise is to reflect on your own natural tendencies so you can better understand how they interact with your child's temperament.

EXTRAVERSION

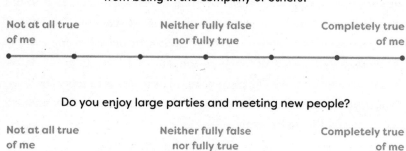

Are you someone who gets energy from being in the company of others?

Not at all true of me — Neither fully false nor fully true — Completely true of me

Do you enjoy large parties and meeting new people?

Not at all true of me — Neither fully false nor fully true — Completely true of me

Are you someone who is talkative and full of energy?

Not at all true of me — Neither fully false nor fully true — Completely true of me

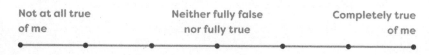

Are you someone who is outgoing and sociable?

Not at all true of me — Neither fully false nor fully true — Completely true of me

All of the above are indicators of Extraversion. Answers on the true side are indicators of higher Extraversion. Answers on the false side suggest that you are lower on Extraversion. Below are some additional indicators of lower Extraversion (i.e. these are coded in the opposite direction).

Are you generally a reserved person?

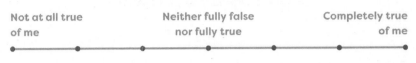

**Do you prefer quiet activities,
like reading a good book, over loud, boisterous parties?**

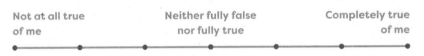

**Do you prefer spending time alone, or with a small number of
close friends, rather than being in a larger group?**

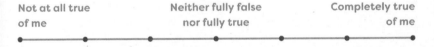

Answers in the positive direction to the above questions, along with answers in the false direction to the first set of questions, are indicators of low Extraversion.

Look back at your answers to the above questions about high Extraversion, and the additional indicators of low Extraversion. Where do most of your marks fall? Overall, where do you fall on Extraversion?

EMOTIONALITY

Are you someone who gets nervous easily?

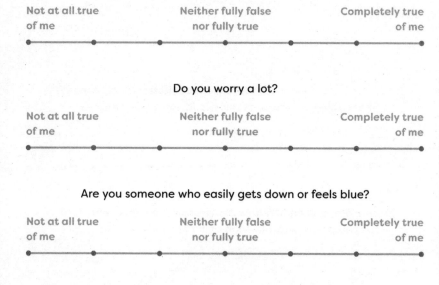

Not at all true of me   Neither fully false nor fully true   Completely true of me

Do you worry a lot?

Not at all true of me   Neither fully false nor fully true   Completely true of me

Are you someone who easily gets down or feels blue?

Not at all true of me   Neither fully false nor fully true   Completely true of me

Do you get very frustrated or upset when things don't go as planned?

Not at all true of me   Neither fully false nor fully true   Completely true of me

Answers in the "true" direction on the above questions are all indicators of higher Emotionality. The following are some additional indicators of low Emotionality.

Are you someone who easily handles stress?

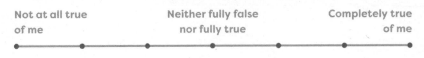

Not at all true of me	Neither fully false nor fully true	Completely true of me

Are you someone whose emotions are usually pretty steady; you don't get easily upset?

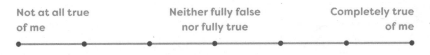

Not at all true of me	Neither fully false nor fully true	Completely true of me

Do you remain calm in tense situations?

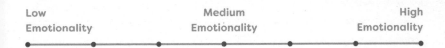

Not at all true of me	Neither fully false nor fully true	Completely true of me

Look back at your answers to the earlier questions about high and low Emotionality. Where do most of your marks fall? Overall, where do you fall on Emotionality?

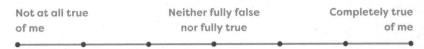

Low Emotionality	Medium Emotionality	High Emotionality

EFFORTFUL CONTROL

Are you good at making a plan and following through?

Not at all true
of me

Neither fully false
nor fully true

Completely true
of me

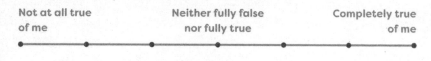

Are you good at persevering at a task until it is finished, even if it is boring?

Not at all true
of me

Neither fully false
nor fully true

Completely true
of me

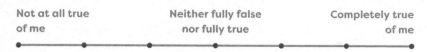

Do you think about things carefully before you do them?

Not at all true
of me

Neither fully false
nor fully true

Completely true
of me

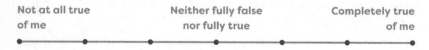

Answers in the true direction to these questions indicate higher levels of Effortful Control. The questions that follow are indicators of lower Effortful Control; answers in the true direction indicate lower levels of Effortful Control.

Are you careless or disorganised?

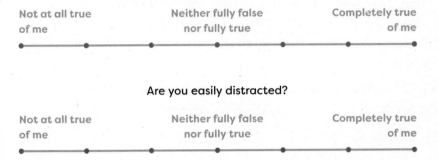

Are you easily distracted?

Look back at your answers to the questions indicating characteristics that represent higher and lower levels of Effortful Control. Where do most of your marks fall? Overall, where do you fall on Effortful Control?

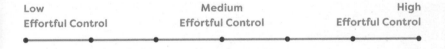

Risk-Taking

There's one more dimension that is important to consider: risk-taking. In children, risk-taking is related to Extraversion and Effortful Control. In adults, with our more complicated and further differentiated brains, we can separate out Risk-Taking from Extraversion and Effortful Control. Take a minute to think about how the following statements relate to you:

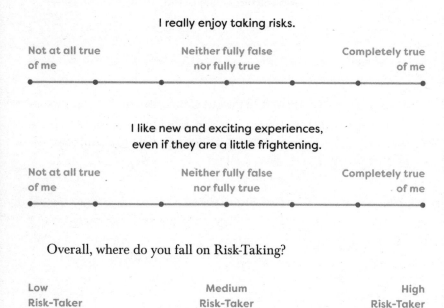

I really enjoy taking risks.

Not at all true of me   Neither fully false nor fully true   Completely true of me

I like new and exciting experiences, even if they are a little frightening.

Not at all true of me   Neither fully false nor fully true   Completely true of me

Overall, where do you fall on Risk-Taking?

Low Risk-Taker   Medium Risk-Taker   High Risk-Taker

My Profile

Based on your responses above, indicate below whether you are Low, Medium, or High on each of the Big Three dimensions, along with Risk-Taking:

DIMENSIONS	MY PROFILE	MY CHILD'S PROFILE
Extraversion (Ex):	Low/Medium/High	Low/Medium/High
Emotionality (Em):	Low/Medium/High	Low/Medium/High
Effortful Control (Ef):	Low/Medium/High	Low/Medium/High
Risk-Taking	Low/Medium/High	

Now look back at your child's profile and compare it to yours. How similar in temperament are you and your child? Many of the stressors that we experience as parents arise from mismatches between our child's natural temperament and the environments that we are creating for our children, which are often unconscious reflections of our own temperaments. The good news is that by understanding and recognising these tension points, many of them can be easily eliminated. Further, by helping your child understand their genetically influenced temperament, you can help them better understand themselves and teach them how to manage their natural tendencies. This will allow them to build their strengths and develop strategies to help them manage situations that are likely to be challenging for them. The next several chapters will discuss each temperament dimension in more detail, and show you how to create a Goodness of Fit for you and your child.

Takeaways

- There are three overarching genetically influenced dimensions (the Three Es) that children differ on: Extraversion (Ex), Emotionality (Em), and Effortful Control (Ef).

- *Extraversion* in children is related to their natural tendencies towards positive affect, activity level, and exploratory behaviour.

- *Emotionality* refers to children's natural tendencies towards distress, fear, and frustration.

- *Effortful Control* refers to how well children can regulate their emotions and behaviour.

- Children with different dispositional styles will present different challenges for parents and have different needs.

- *Goodness of Fit* refers to the match between children and their parents, as well as their environment more broadly.

- Children thrive when there is a match between their temperaments and their environment.

- Understanding your child's natural dispositional styles—and your own—can help you provide Goodness of Fit for your child, reducing everyone's stress.

CHAPTER 4

· · · ▬ · · ·

Extraversion:
The "Ex" Factor

Are you an extravert or an introvert?

Virtually all of us have a ready answer to that. I'm an extravert. My idea of a fun Friday night is getting together with a big group of girlfriends for a night of dinner and drinks (and back in my twenties, dancing!) at a trendy new restaurant. I love being around people; I love going to new places, trying new things. If I'm cooped up at home too long without human interaction, I start to go stir-crazy. When my poor husband walks in the door after I've spent all day writing (read: at home in front of my computer by myself), he can barely make it inside before I start peppering him with questions.

We talk a lot about extraversion and introversion in adults. Tell an introvert that they have to spend their Friday night at an office party making small talk with strangers and they'll cringe. Put an extravert behind a desk all day with no one to talk to and they'll be miserable. In adults, we recognise the many ways that our level of extraversion influences our day-to-day lives, the way we respond to others, and the activities we choose (or avoid!). But we don't thoughtfully consider the impact of extraversion/introversion nearly as much in our children, and that's a mistake.

Children show natural preferences at a young age for being around other people, and how much they like boisterous versus quiet activities. Just as with adults, trying to force them into environments that aren't a good fit can lead to profound discomfort. But even worse—children don't have the cognitive maturity to deal with that discomfort, which can lead to temper tantrums or embarrassing behaviour.

In this chapter, we'll talk about what to expect from children who are High to Low on Extraversion. It will help you better understand your child, and how their level of extraversion impacts their behaviour and your interactions with them. We'll talk about the good things and not-so-good things associated with different levels of extraversion. Finally, we'll talk about the parenting strategies that are most important for kids with different degrees of extraversion.

Although we talk about extraversion and introversion as if they are two different things, remember that in actuality it's a continuum. In the research world, we say that people vary from high to low on Extraversion. In this chapter, I'll use "extravert" and "introvert" as shorthand for kids who are at the high and low ends of the continuum, but it's important to remember that children are not necessarily "either/or"; they vary across the full spectrum, with many of them falling somewhere in the middle. These medium Extraversion children may display some characteristics typical of extraverts and some characteristics more typical of introverts, just as is true for adults.

The High Ex Child

My three-year-old was sitting at the edge of the toddler pool when another young girl about his age walked over and sat down next to him. "Hi, I'm Savannah, what's your name? I think we're going to be friends. Don't you just love the pool? I have a pool at my house too. Maybe you can come over to my house one day. That would be fun! Let's ask our parents. We could play house too. You could be the daddy and I'll be the mummy. I have lots of toys. What kind of toys do you like?" My son sat there quietly staring at her as if she was a foreign being dropped in from an alien planet. Savannah is the consummate High Ex child, and my little introvert had no idea what to do with her!

Children who are high on Extraversion naturally enjoy meeting new people, going new places, and trying new things. They are energized by being around others. They will strike up conversations with strangers. They can be talkative (my nickname growing up was Tilly the Talker; my mum's was Last Word Lynn—a clear example of High Ex running in a family). High Ex children tend to think out loud; they like to tell you all about their day and the many thoughts running through their brains. They like a wide variety of activities and people. They are comfortable being the centre of attention, and often will seek it out.

The Good

If you're the parent of a High Ex child, you've probably already discovered there are a number of great things that come with extraversion. High Ex children are more socially active; they are quicker to make new friends. Take a High Ex child to the playground and they will run right over and start playing with the other kids. If a pickup basketball game forms in the neighbourhood, they'll jump right in.

High Ex children can be charming. It's sweet to see your child interact with others. I remember watching my nephew Greyson toddle his tiny three-year-old self over to a group of older children throwing a ball at the beach and say, "Hi, guys, can I play?!" He was so adorable that the group of mostly older girls took right to him for the day (and Greyson's mum got a brief respite from running after him!). The ease with which High Ex children interact with others often endears them to both adults and other children alike.

This willingness to meet new people and try new things also provides a lot of opportunity for growth and learning for your child. Increased interactions with other children and adults promotes social skills. A willingness to go new places gives them more opportunity to experience and learn from the world. Interacting with others and trying new things produce positive emotions in High Ex individuals; it has been suggested that this positive feedback loop can create greater motivation to achieve goals. Their natural tendency towards positive emotion may also serve as a buffer against challenging experiences.

Extraversion can lead to advantages at school, and eventually in the workplace, as extraverts are often perceived as natural leaders. As a society, we tend to value the characteristics typical of extraverts. This has been called the *Extravert Advantage*. New research suggests that one unexpected way extraverts may get an edge is by being better at unconsciously copying the body language, speech patterns, and movements of the people they interact with. This has been called *mimicry* and could result from being more attentive to other people. The matching of speech and body language is known to increase positive feelings between people, and it may contribute to why people seem to be more drawn to extraverts.

The Not-So-Good

There are a lot of great things that come with having a High Ex child . . . but there are also some not-so-great things. High Ex children tend to be always "on the go". Their desire for activity and excitement can translate into a lot of unbridled energy! For us parents, that means we have to keep them busy. All that activity can be exhausting, especially if you are lower on Extraversion. Many High Ex children are also Low Ef (Effortful Control). Low self-control combined with lots of energy can be a recipe for things getting broken around the house! One of my friends used to joke that she never knew so many parents were out and about at the break of day until she had her second (High Ex) child. With her first (Low Ex) child, she had developed a morning routine that involved her enjoying a cup of coffee while her child played with her toys nearby, building with Legos, doing puzzles. With child number two, there were no more quiet relaxing Saturday mornings; it was chaos from the time her child's eyes opened and feet hit the ground!

Another challenge is that because High Ex children crave constant interaction with other people—let's be honest—they can sometimes be trying. High Ex children only know their own way of being in the world (just like all of us), so they can lack self-awareness. They may fail to realise that not everyone wants company all the time, whether it's other children or the adults in their life. High Ex children will follow you into the bathroom, your bedroom, around the house. As my husband still needs to remind me, not everyone finds constant conversation invigorating.

If you're the parent of a High Ex child, there's something else you need to have on your radar: your social small child may be adorable, but your High Ex teenager may be a royal pain. High Ex children are more likely to pose a number of challenges to parents as they get older. Because they love to be around their peers, High Ex adolescents and young adults are more susceptible to peer influence. Their social nature makes them care more about what others think. As adolescents, they are more likely to use alcohol or other drugs, and engage in other risky behaviours. The toddler who is adorably entertaining your friends now with their rendition of Beyoncé's latest hit is also more likely to be dancing on tables at a freshers' party in fifteen years.

The Low Ex Child

My stepdaughter would play in the house all day long if we let her. She pulls out her little dishes and we play kitchen for a while. Then she plays with her dolls. She'll take out a book and sit in her reading chair and look at the pictures. Then she colours, or does a puzzle. She plays with her little ponies and builds a whole imaginary world for them.

My husband and I are good for about ten minutes of playing kitchen or ponies before we want to pull out our hair.

Children who are low in Extraversion are more involved in their own internal worlds of ideas, emotions, and play. Low Ex children enjoy quiet time alone. They don't need a constant flurry of activities, adventures, or other people. In fact, too much stimulation can feel overwhelming to the Low Ex child. When they are around lots of people or engaged in a busy activity, they need quiet time afterward to recharge. Low Ex children prefer to spend time with a small number of people rather than big groups. They don't like being the centre of attention and they are slower to warm up to new people. Whereas High Ex children may have wide social circles and a wide array of interests, Low Ex children prefer a smaller number of close friends and enjoy concentrating on a single activity. When they are comfortable with you, or really excited about a topic, however, they can be very open and chatty, which may lead you to wonder what happened to the charming child you know when they are around other people and suddenly go mute. Low Ex children like to observe first before entering a new activity or group. They need to be encouraged to share their opinions or to speak up.

The Good

Despite all the talk of the "Extravert Advantage," there are a lot of great things that come with being low on Extraversion. Low Ex children can be lower maintenance (especially if they are not high on Emotionality). They are more naturally inclined to respect the space of others (read: you might still get some alone time as a parent!). They tend to be not as clingy or as likely to be overly boisterous at school. They are less influenced by trends and peers, and more likely to adopt their own perspectives and ideas. They tend to think more deeply about things before making a decision or jumping to action. The physicist Albert Einstein was famous for his introversion; he once stated, "The monotony and solitude of a quiet life stimulates the creative mind". Introverts are often creative, thoughtful, and more intentional. They tend to cultivate deep connections with people; they prefer quality over quantity. Their tendency to be more private is also more likely to build independence.

The Not-So-Good

Children who are low in Extraversion are more likely to need to be coaxed to try new things. They like their comfort zones, and new people or places can be exhausting for them. So without a little push, the Low Ex child may not want to explore the unknown or meet new people. Social situations can be stressful for them. If they are high on Emotionality, putting them in situations where they are uncomfortable can lead to temper tantrums or outbursts. Because being around other people is more draining for them, Low Ex children also need more downtime after activities, or breaks from the action. Without enough quiet time, they are likely to get irritable or cranky.

Because they are quieter, Low Ex children also risk being overlooked. They don't command the attention that their High Ex peers do, and they are less likely to speak up. Because they are less likely to engage with their parents or teachers, it can give the impression that they don't need them as much. This can mean that Low Ex children don't get the attention they need and deserve from the important adults in their lives. The fact that they are more independent and more likely to think for themselves can also make them less susceptible to outside influence—that's great when it comes to peer pressure, but not so great when they are less inclined to follow your directives. Because introverts are more content in their own thoughts, and can take longer to respond to you, they may come across as stubborn. In situations where Low Ex children are pressured to speak up, or make quick decisions, they can feel stressed or freeze up. This can lead to the misperception that Low Ex children are being obstinate, or are not as bright or quick as their more extraverted peers. It may also lead them to question whether they are as likeable or smart as other children, or whether there is something wrong with them.

Low Ex versus Shy

Low Ex children are sometimes described as shy, but shyness and introversion are actually different things. The reason these two traits are confused is because low Extraversion and shyness can lead to similar behaviours, such as reluctance to join in group activities or play with other children. The primary difference is that Low Ex children *enjoy* being by themselves and have a preference for small groups. Shy children want to be part of the group, but are nervous (or at the extreme, socially anxious) about socialising. Shy children can fall anywhere on the Extraversion dimension. When they are medium to high on Extraversion, their nervousness about interacting with other children can lead to loneliness because their preference would be to be around others. Low Ex children, by contrast, may have no problem interacting with other children, they just choose not to. As a parent, you're in the best position to figure out whether your child is Low Ex or shy. Ask yourself: do they seem unhappy being by themselves? Do they want to be around other children, but are too anxious to join in? If the answer to either of those questions is yes, then your child may be shy rather than introverted and can benefit from working on their social skills. While shyness is partly genetically influenced (most everything is), it is not a temperamental trait per se, and is definitely something you can work on with your child.

Strategies for Growing Your Child's Social Skills

Whether you have a High Ex child who constantly talks over others or a Low Ex child who has trouble joining in group activities, most children benefit from honing their social skills. Just like walking and talking, interacting with others is something that is learned and fine-tuned through practice. Social skills can be pretty nuanced for a developing brain; for example, there are times when you want your child to speak up (e.g. if they see a friend being teased), and times when you hope they will keep their mouth shut (e.g. when they feel compelled to comment on the person in line next to you at the supermarket: "Mummy, that lady has crazy hair!").

The good news is that children are constantly refining their social skills as they grow (often adults are too). One of the best ways you can help your child develop social acumen is by *teaching through conversation*. Emotional competence is central to most social situations, meaning that children interact better with others when they have an understanding of how emotions connect to behaviour. There are opportunities for teaching these skills everywhere (just ask my son; he calls them "mum tips", though now, at age thirteen, he says that with an eye roll). For example, you can read a book with your child and talk about what happened—connecting emotions to the characters' behaviour. Why do you think the bunny got so upset? How do you think the piggy felt when the elephant took the toy away? When your child talks to you about something another child did at school (usually this was my child reporting on another child's misbehaviour: "Guess what David did today?!"), you can use it as an opportunity to talk about making different choices.

You can also role-play areas where your child is struggling with social situations. For example, if your Low Ex child has trouble looking adults in the eye when speaking, you can practise together, and help them understand why the skill is important. Tell your child a story while looking at the ground and then ask how it made them feel. That will help your child understand that it is uncomfortable for the other person when someone talks without making eye contact. Then have your child practise telling you a story while holding eye contact with you.

"Practice makes perfect" (or at least better) isn't just for team sports; it is equally applicable when it comes to children's social skills. Make sure to praise your child when they handle a situation well—when your High Ex child gives others a turn to speak, when your Low Ex child takes the initiative to make a new friend. Verbally rewarding child behaviour is a great way to help your child learn, and to increase the frequency of behaviours you want to see more of (more on this in the next chapter).

THE HIGH EX CHILD	THE LOW EX CHILD
Enjoys meeting new people	Prefers smaller groups and close friends
Likes going to new places	Needs time to recharge after social activities
Enjoys trying new things	Likes to observe before starting an activity
Is talkative, thinks out loud	Enjoys quiet activities
Likes being the centre of attention	Doesn't like being the centre of attention
Makes new friends easily	Is slow to warm up to people
Needs lots of approval	Is content playing alone

Parenting to Your Child's Extraversion Level

Figuring out what our children need can feel like one of the most challenging parts of parenting; fortunately, knowing where your child falls on Extraversion can be a big help. Children at different levels of Extraversion need different things from their parents. As parents, we can make easy adjustments to create a better Goodness of Fit for our children and decrease challenging behaviour. Children with different levels of Extraversion also have different *areas for growth* that may not come naturally to them, but that we can help them develop.

Parenting the High Ex Child

High Ex children crave interaction—from you and from others. Here are some strategies for giving them the outlets they need and the attention they desire, while also teaching them that quiet time is not a bad thing, and that they need to learn to share the limelight.

Give them lots of social stimulation. Children who are high on Extraversion tend to thrive in active, busy environments. They need opportunities to socialise. As the parent of a High Ex child, you can expose them to many different environments because they are more open to trying new things, and more likely to enjoy them. Playdates, amusement parks, bowling alleys, concerts, sporting events, children's theatre, dance/gym classes, camps/group activities, parks—anywhere that is people-centric is likely to be a good fit for your High Ex child. Look into the activities available in your local area. You may want to make a list and post it on your refrigerator. One friend had a list of all the children's activities (museums, parks, etc.) in our area posted on the wall next to her breakfast table, along with the daily hours for each. She knew exactly what parks opened at what time on what days so she could quickly whisk her High Ex son out the door after breakfast before all that energy started bouncing off the walls of her small terraced house.

Provide lots of feedback. High Ex children like to talk things through. Their brains are programmed for interaction. They get energy and motivation from getting positive responses from others. That means your High Ex child craves your attention and input. They want you to watch them as they climb the monkey bars and tell them how high they are. They want to tell you all about what they did at school that day and have you get excited about it with them. If you are also High Ex, this likely comes naturally to you: "Wow, look at you on top of the monkey bars!" "Oh gosh, that sounds like so much fun!" If you are Low Ex, it probably won't feel nearly as comfortable. I've had Low Ex parents tell me that they feel ridiculous constantly commenting on their child's behaviour, or that they don't feel like it's good for a child to get constant praise.

If you're a Low Ex parent, try to remember that your High Ex child's brain is wired differently and that they need feedback to help them grow. If they don't get it from you, they will seek it out from others—which may not always be a good thing. Note that giving your child feedback does not mean showering them with false praise; you can just reflect back their behaviour: "Sounds like you had a big day at school!" "You played so much with the other kids!" But don't be afraid to celebrate their achievements as well: "You are riding your bike so well!" "You have really learned how to play nicely with others." Providing positive feedback is a great way to reinforce the behaviours you want to see more of in your children. And you don't want to ignore the good and comment only on the bad, as your child will quickly discover what kind of behaviour elicits your attention!

Teach them to slow down. Because High Ex children want to be constantly on the go, it's up to you to teach them the importance of slowing down. Yes, there are many wonderful things associated with exploring the world and getting involved in lots of activities, but all of us need to recharge, whether we realise it or not. This doesn't come naturally to High Ex children. High Ex children, especially as they get older, can overextend themselves in their excitement to be involved in many activities. This can lead them to feel overwhelmed. As the parent of a High Ex child, you can start to teach them from an early age the importance of taking some downtime. Learning how to regulate themselves so they don't overdo it is an important skill for High Ex children to develop. Though High Ex children like social interaction and the positive feelings that come with it, they can still wear themselves down and get overtired, leading to whining, arguing, or temper tantrums. None of us is our best self when we're tired.

Make a point to find time in between social activities or outings to do quieter activities. Importantly, talk to your child about why you are doing this, so they understand and start to internalise the importance of taking time to relax and refresh. Here are some suggestions for what that might look like:

HIGH EX CHILD: "Let's go to the pool!"

PARENT: "We already spent the morning at the park with friends, and I know you love being around other people, but all of us need some time to recharge. How about you and me do a puzzle together instead?"

. . .

HIGH EX CHILD: "I want to go to the park!"

PARENT: "I know it's fun to be out and about a lot of the time, but we all need to slow down and take some time for ourselves or else we can wear ourselves out. Why don't you work on building that new Lego ship you got for your birthday?"

Don't be surprised if your High Ex child resists or protests. After all, their natural tendency is to want to be on the go! Our brains are wired to want more of the things we like, and High Ex children find interaction rewarding. But part of our role as parents is to gently challenge our children's natural tendencies to help them realise that we have to regulate our desires. And as the parent, you are the best gauge of how much activity and interaction your child needs, and how much they can handle. By that, I mean you don't have to be rigid about having downtime for a set period of time every day (unless that works well for you and your child). You can get a sense of how much activity is the right amount for your child and work in downtime accordingly. For some children it may be once a day, for others it may be once a week. The important thing is that you talk with them about the need to slow down and learn to enjoy time to themselves. Help them start to see that some quiet time can be rewarding too. Say "Did you notice how energised you felt after you took some quiet time to read in your room? Now you're ready to go again!" Or "Sometimes when we're constantly on the go, we start to feel too revved up. It's like how when a pot of water gets too hot it starts to boil over! So we just turn down the heat, and do something calmer for a little while."

When you find your High Ex child enjoying a quieter activity, make sure you point it out and encourage them so they can start to make the connection: "What an amazing puzzle you put together! You seem really proud. It feels good to work on projects on your own sometimes." Or "It's nice to just lie on the grass and look at the clouds for a little while after a busy morning." Over time it will become a habit that they more naturally fit in to their days.

Teach them to reflect and empathise. Your High Ex child may need you to help them learn to be more reflective. As we discussed above, we only know our own way of being in the world. And it's a natural tendency to assume others think the way that we do. Help your High Ex child understand that while they are energized by people and activity and conversation, not everyone is. Some people need more quiet time to process their thoughts, or enjoy being around other people without so much conversation. If they have a sibling or friend who you recognise is lower on Extraversion, you can use that person as an example to help them understand: "You know your friend Michael? You have so much fun playing together, but have you noticed that Michael is much quieter than you? Sometimes you need to pause to make sure Michael has time to talk too." Or "I know you like to process things by thinking out loud, but sometimes it's good to stop and think about things first." Chapter 6 on Effortful Control has lots of strategies for teaching your child to slow down and think before acting. You may find some of these helpful for your High Ex child.

Parenting the Low Ex Child

Low Ex children don't demand our attention the way that High Ex children do. But that doesn't mean they don't have needs too. Here are some strategies you can implement if you are the parent of a Low Ex child, to help your quieter child thrive.

Help them feel loved and accepted. This may seem like a no-brainer. Of course we want our children to feel loved and accepted. But the reality is that we live in an extravert's world. I've read that extraverts outnumber introverts three to one. We are a culture that admires rugged individualism, getting out and doing things, speaking your mind. We live in a society constructed by extraverts. Because of this, Low Ex children can feel out of place, "lesser", or like they don't fit in. Depending on the temperaments of the other adults and children in your household, they may feel this way at home. They are also likely to feel this way at school, where children who speak up and volunteer (usually High Ex children) often stand out more. Young children may not understand why they feel out of place.

One of the most important things you can do as a parent is to help your Low Ex child understand himself. Help him understand that there is nothing wrong with him. Talk to your child about how we are all born with different temperaments. Tell them that some children love to be surrounded by other people and activities, and other children feel more comfortable in quiet activities or on their own. Then ask them which one sounds more like them. Explain that they are more introverted (I use this language with children, as they are likely to encounter it in the world, and so it's helpful for them to understand the term). Help them understand all the things that are wonderful about introverts—they are more quiet thinkers, that quiet time allows for more creativity and deep thought. That they make great friends because they form deep connections. Search on the Internet together for famous introverts so that they understand you can be successful as an introvert and that their disposition is special.

Because we live in an extravert's world, your Low Ex child may need more support and encouragement from you. They need to know that you love them even though they aren't always the centre of attention or the most popular child on the playground. If they struggle with their peers because they are "too quiet," and hence don't feel accepted, work with them on the social skills strategies discussed above. Low Ex children need to understand that more isn't always better, that little things are "enough"—snuggling with you, reading a book, playing together at the house, a few close friends. Your Low Ex child is more likely to enjoy the simple pleasures in life, and as their parent, you can help them see that as a gift rather than a liability.

Find activities that are a good fit for their disposition. Low Ex children naturally enjoy activities that involve fewer people and that don't overwhelm them with social stimulation. Building with Legos (or as they get older, model planes or ships), reading, doing puzzles, colouring, playing with toys in their room: give your Low Ex child plenty of options that are individual ways to express their creativity. Other choices that are good for Low Ex children include a trip to the library, or an art museum, or staying home to watch a movie together. There are lots of great sports options that are good for Low Ex children as well. Think golf, tennis, ice skating, rowing, rock climbing, biking—sports that are more individual. These are all great ways to get them active but that do not necessitate their coordinating and working with a big team. Photography is a great hobby for Low Ex children. It allows them to be outside experiencing the world and in the company of others, while still feeling safe and less exposed by being behind a camera. My Low Ex child has always enjoyed being the "photographer" at family events. He can be a part of the group without feeling like he has to be talking with everyone constantly. Other great hobbies for Low Ex children include painting, gardening, or cooking—these are all ways that they can spend time with you, with others, and out in the world, without becoming exhausted by a need for constant social interaction. Also consider getting them involved with animals. Introverts often love the companionship that animals provide; they are less chatty and exhausting than people! Volunteering at a local animal shelter is a great way to get your Low Ex child involved in doing good without needing too much interaction with other people.

Give them a quiet place that is their own. Low Ex children need a space where they can be alone with their thoughts. It could be a bedroom, or if that's not possible in your home, you can get creative. They could have their own little fort, or you could create a corner stuffed with comfy pillows and hidden by a sheet tacked to the wall. The important thing is that they have somewhere that is off-limits to everyone else and that they can feel is their own special place. Low Ex children need a way to retreat into their own world and get away when the world around them is too stimulating. They need time alone to recharge.

Help them recognise when they need quiet time. Some Low Ex children are great at recognising on their own when they need some downtime. When we have people over to the house for dinner or a playdate, my three-year-old Low Ex child will eventually start to get fussy over minor things. It's clear that all the people and activity are just becoming too much. When that happens, she usually looks at us and declares that she needs to go upstairs and "take a little nap". She'll go to her room and look at a book for five to fifteen minutes and return recharged as her delightful little self! Sometimes we recognise she's headed that way and ask, "Do you need a little quiet time?" and she almost always responds affirmatively with relief and heads up to her room for a quick break.

But many Low Ex children need some help recognising when they are becoming overstimulated. You may have to help them learn to take quiet time to recharge after being around other people. Help them identify when they are feeling overwhelmed, and encourage them to find ways to take some time to themselves. For example, if you're at a birthday party and you can tell it is becoming too much, you can say, "Should we go outside and take a break for a few minutes?" Or if the gathering is at your house, you could suggest that they come help you with something in the kitchen. Help your child understand that it's OK to leave for a little bit and then rejoin the fun. It's the child equivalent of the adult taking a break from the cocktail party out on the balcony. Help them recognise how it recharges their battery to get away for a few minutes. You can say, "Whew, it's a lot to be around lots of people. You seem more relaxed after taking a few minutes away". You can also help your child rejoin the fun when they return. "Oh look! Hannah is playing a fun game. Hannah, can you show Josh how it works?" Remember that Low Ex children often like to observe before joining a group, so it's OK if they want to take a few minutes and watch before jumping in.

The Medium Ex Child

My husband calls himself an Extraverted Introvert. Adults who are medium on Extraversion often describe themselves this way. *Ambivert* is another term that is widely used to refer to people who are medium on Extraversion. Medium Extraversion individuals show some characteristics that we associate with Extraversion (High Ex) and some that we associate with introversion (Low Ex). Because most behaviour follows a bell curve pattern in the population, there are actually many people who fall into the Medium Ex range.

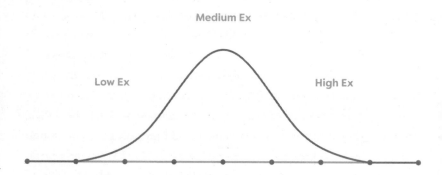

Medium Ex children enjoy being around other people and trying new things *to an extent*, but they also enjoy quieter activities and need some downtime to recharge as well. If you have a Medium Ex child, you probably see elements of them in the descriptions of the High *and* Low Ex children. Since your child is not as extreme in either direction with respect to their natural Extraversion tendencies, they are likely to enjoy a mixture of the recommended activities for High and Low Ex children. The key for you is figuring out your child's patterns: how much activity that is high in social interaction is right for your child? How much downtime do they need? By observing your child over time, you will get a sense of this. It may happen without requiring much attention from you. Since Medium Ex children enjoy both High and Low Ex activities, they can be more adaptable, especially if they are low on Emotionality. But if you find that your child is getting cranky when you are doing particular activities, it may be worth keeping a journal for a week. Write down the times you spend in different types of activities each day and how each activity went. For example, one entry might look like this:

Saturday:

- **8–10 a.m.:** playgroup at the park with three other friends (happy, had lots of fun)
- **10 a.m.–noon:** children's museum (happy, lots of fun)
- lunch, nap
- **2–4 p.m.:** older sibling's football match (very grumpy, misbehaved)

It's possible that your child just finds football boring, but it's also possible that they were tuckered out from a morning full of activities. Keeping a journal for a week or more will help you differentiate these possibilities. If you start to see a repeated pattern whereby your child is getting cranky or misbehaving after long stretches of social outings, you could try building in more quiet activities to give them some downtime in between. For example, if you know that their older sibling has a match in the afternoon, you may try doing some quiet playtime at the house after the morning playdate so that they have time to recharge and will be excited to run around at the game again in the afternoon. If the pattern is that they're only grumpy at football matches, well, you have your answer there too.

Depending on whether they lean more towards the High Ex end or towards the Low Ex end (and depending on the Extraversion profile of other members of your family), your Medium Ex child may need help with developing certain skills described in either the High or Low Ex profiles. For example, if you notice that your Medium Ex child is starting to command the dinner table and their Low Ex sibling isn't getting a word in, then you can work with your Medium Ex child on making sure to allow everyone a chance to speak. Conversely, if you notice your Medium Ex child has been constantly on the go keeping up with their High Ex sibling, then you may need to help them recognise when they need to take a break. The more time you spend with your child, the more insight you'll have into whether your child needs a little help in any of the areas described above. But in general, because they are not as extreme, Medium Ex children are often more "go with the flow," enjoying a mixture of activities and understanding the perspectives of their more High and Low Ex peers.

SUGGESTED ACTIVITIES FOR . . .	
THE HIGH EX CHILD	**THE LOW EX CHILD**
Playgroups	Reading
Parks with lots of children	Puzzles
Bowling	Photography
Dance/gym classes	Library
Children's concerts	Lego
Sporting events	Playing in their room
Children's theatre	Colouring
Camps/group activities	Movie night in
Children's museums	Art museums
Team sports	Individual sports
Amusement parks	Gardening
Zoo	Cooking

Note: Low Ex children and High Ex children are likely to enjoy activities from each list, but High Ex children need more social stimulation and Low Ex children need more quiet activities.

Challenging Their Extraversion Level

The parenting strategies above are all ways to create Goodness of Fit with your High to Low Ex child. They will allow you to better match your child's environment with their natural tendencies to reduce challenging behaviour. Maybe you find yourself thinking (or maybe your spouse has argued), "But that's not the way the world works! The world does not bend to a person's every need, and our children need to learn that". It's a fair point. I am not suggesting that you keep your Low Ex child playing happily in their room and never expose them to other children, or that you have to be carting your High Ex child all over town to a million activities and events. Understanding their natural tendencies will help you understand the environments that are likely to be good fits, and the environments that are likely to be challenging for your child. Some of that is within your control as a parent, so you can use that knowledge to reduce, or at least demystify, the times when your child gets upset or acts out.

But understanding their temperament does not make you a slave to them! All of us have to be in environments that are outside our comfort zones. High Ex children have to learn how to be alone sometimes, and Low Ex children have to be able to survive in a social setting. Understanding what situations are likely to be challenging for your child doesn't mean you have to avoid them; it empowers you to better anticipate and prepare for them.

Let's be honest: challenging your child's natural tendencies can be . . . well, challenging. When children are in environments that don't align well with their natural tendencies, it creates a mismatch. Mismatches cause stress. Children react to this stress in different ways, which is related to where they fall on Emotionality. How well your child handles the stress that results from a mismatch between their environment and their natural tendency will influence how much you can push them. Highly emotional children have a lot more difficulty managing a mismatch between their environment and their Extraversion. Both of my children are low on Extraversion (the irony) but they differ on their Emotionality. My son is Low Ex-High Em. My stepdaughter is Low Ex-Low Em. Both of them naturally tend towards preferring time playing alone, or with a parent or small number of friends. Put them in a big group of children and they will clam up and stay on the sidelines and watch. But my son's high Emotionality led him to get really upset when he was put in a situation that made him uncomfortable. This was abundantly clear in how he responded to some of his early birthday parties. As someone who is High Ex, I love a big gathering, and so for my son's second and third birthdays I threw him a large party and invited lots of friends—of both the toddler and adult variety. For two years in a row, we sang "Happy Birthday" and he freaked out, crawling under the table one year and behind a sofa the next. My guests were left awkwardly finishing the song while I tried to coax him out. For him, being the centre of attention in a crowd was just too much to bear. Eventually I figured this out, gave up my aspiration to host large theme-based birthday parties, and we now do small birthday celebrations with the family or a couple of his close friends.

Because I'm a slow learner (or glutton for punishment), I reverted back to my party-planning ways with my stepdaughter and we threw a large barnyard birthday party for her third birthday, complete with a full petting zoo in our urban back garden. Although she is Low Ex, my stepdaughter is low on Emotionality, so she was able to handle the (literal) zoo. She quietly observed the chaos of children running loose with goats and sheep, and found a bunny off on the side to pet. She looked slightly uncomfortable when everyone gathered around the barn cake to sing and had to be encouraged to blow out the candles, but she didn't disappear under the furniture in tears. Because she is better able to manage her distress, we are able to expose her to more "mismatched" situations without it resulting in total disaster.

So what to do when there is a mismatch between temperament and environment and your child is prone to distress? The choice is up to you: abort or prepare.

Sometimes you may decide it's just not worth it. Do you really need to be at the launch of the new children's museum, or could you wait a couple weeks and check it out with your child when it won't be as packed? Is attending the neighbour child's birthday bash really worth the potential meltdown? If you don't care that much, or if your child is having a bad day (or if you are!), you may decide that you just can't handle it. *And that's OK.* The world will not stop revolving because you didn't make it to little Isabela's fourth birthday party.

But sometimes it is worth it. It is an event that is important to you, or that you think is important for your child to attend, whether they like it or not. If that is the case, then the key is to *prepare.* Do not just assume that you can spring the family reunion on your Low Ex child and they will somehow be fine with a bunch of distant aunts and third cousins they've never met fawning all over them. Do not tell your High Ex child on the way to the library that they will need to sit quietly for hours while you get some work done. Talk to your child beforehand (and by "beforehand" I do not mean as you are getting into the car to leave). Let them know about the upcoming event. Talk with them about their feelings. Then work together to develop a plan. Here's what this might look like:

PARENT: "Alyssa, on Saturday, we have a family reunion. Do you know what a family reunion is?"

LOW EX CHILD: "No."

PARENT: "It's when a big group of people who are all related get together. Kind of like when we get together with Grandma and Grandpa and Aunt B's family, but with lots more people."

LOW EX CHILD *(looking sceptical)*: "Lots of people I don't know?"

PARENT: "There will be a lot of new people there. How does that make you feel?"

LOW EX CHILD: "I don't want to go. You know I don't like being around lots of people."

PARENT: "I know it's not your favourite thing to do, and that it can feel overwhelming. But it's important that we go. Let's come up with strategies that you can use if it starts to feel like too much. Do you have any ideas?"

Depending on the age and maturity of your child, they may or may not be able to generate a plan. Brainstorm with them. "If you start to feel overwhelmed, maybe you could go outside and explore the back garden for a while? Or maybe you could go upstairs and play with Grandma's cat?" Let your child know that it's OK for them to take a break if they need to. Help them come up with a strategy.

Preparation doesn't stop at preparing your child, it also means preparing yourself. When your reserves are low—perhaps you got a poor night's sleep, or have other stressors going on in your life, or you just don't have the energy for it—it might not be the best time to challenge a trait. For the family reunion, bowing out might not be an option, but for some events (probably more than you think) you can always abort if it looks like you or your child just aren't up to the task. The reality is that even with the best planning and preparation, sometimes a child just won't be able to cope, especially if they are high on Emotionality (more on that in the next chapter). And as the parent, you need to be able to take a deep breath and reset. You need to think through how you will handle the situation if your child can't rise to the occasion. You need to have a plan of your own in case your child just can't overcome their distress.

I will confess that this has always been the hardest part for me. I hate it when I've done everything I'm supposed to—talked to my child, come up with a plan, practised what he would say and do—and yet when the time came . . . he just couldn't do it, whether that meant a melt-down or just a staunch refusal to participate. It's frustrating because no matter how much you prepare, a part of it is out of your control. I paid for many a summer camp that my child said he wanted to do, we talked about it, prepared for it, and yet at drop-off when he saw the group of children, he froze and refused to get out of the car. Never mind that we had a plan. Never mind that I'd prepaid for a week of toddler all-sport fun. Never mind that I had a meeting to get to right after drop-off. Never mind that we both felt great about being prepared to have it go smoothly. In the moment, he couldn't do it. And that's when, as the parent, I had to revert to *my* preparation. Because as frustrated as I was, as much as I wanted to scream at him that *we had a plan*, and he was going to be fine so just get out of the car so I could get to work!—that was the moment when I had to remember my preparation: take a deep breath, stay calm, and talk through it one more time. Sometimes he calmed down and came around and headed in to camp. And sometimes he didn't. So we would try again another day. In the moment, it makes you want to pull your hair out. But I can tell you that at age thirteen he jumps out of the car to head over to his friends as fast as possible. Hang in there. It's a marathon, not a sprint. Keep on trying and your efforts will eventually help your child gain the skills they need to manage their temperament.

How Your Level of Extraversion Affects Your Parenting

Before you had a child, you probably imagined all the fun things you would do together. And the activities you imagined, whether you realised it or not, were likely related to your own level of Extraversion. High Ex parents can't wait to take their children to the zoo, the park, to do play-dates with their other friends (and throw their kids huge birthday parties). Low Ex parents look forward to quality time with their child reading books, doing art projects. The world we imagine creating for our child is a product of our own temperament and interests. And when you luck out and have a match between your Extraversion and your child's

Extraversion, it works great! High Ex parents with High Ex children delight in exploring activities and parks and going to social outings. Low Ex parents with Low Ex children enjoy quality time playing together at home or going for walks in nature. These sets of parents and children have a natural Goodness of Fit. But it's also possible that you and your child could have completely different temperaments. Mismatches between children and their parents on Extraversion are often the root of many parental concerns and challenges.

The High Ex Parent with a Low Ex Child

Extraverted parents of introverted children tend to worry a lot. My child is a loner! They aren't going to have friends! They stay in their room too much! They are refusing to participate in the school play! They need to get out and experience the world!

I'm a High Ex parent with two Low Ex children. Trust me, I get it.

But what I've come to appreciate is that Low Ex children *are* experiencing the world, just in a very different way than we extraverts do.* And as hard as it is for us to imagine—it's not a lesser way. It's just different. Low Ex individuals don't need to be surrounded by a whirlwind of activity and people. They like having quality relationships with a small number of people. Usually, within that small circle is us, their parents. When Low Ex children are comfortable, they can be very chatty and delightful. But when in a larger group, they will close up. This can be very puzzling or frustrating for us High Ex parents. Why is my child, who is so fun and delightful with me, being such a dud when around others?! We want our friends and relatives to see the delightful person that we know them to be. We may pressure our child to be "on",

---

* For other High Ex parents trying to better understand the Low Ex experience, I found the book *The Introvert Advantage: How Quiet People Can Thrive in an Extrovert World*, by Marti Olsen Laney, Psy.D., Workman Publishing Company (2002), to be very enlightening and insightful.

to conform to our extraverted world or way of being. I know I have been guilty of this.

But here's what I've learned—from my own introverted children, from talking with other self-proclaimed introverts, and from researching introversion. Sometimes your child just wants alone time. It doesn't mean they won't ever have friends. It doesn't mean that they are destined to live in your basement forever. They just need space to be quiet. They need to process and recharge. Sometimes they will want time away from you; that doesn't mean they don't need you, or love you, or that they never want to be around you. But we High Ex parents can be exhausting for our Low Ex children. Sometimes they just want to sit or play in silence near us. If you ever had a needy boyfriend or girlfriend, you've experienced this: you'd like them more if they were around less! That's how our Low Ex children can feel about us.

The takeaway for us High Ex parents with Low Ex children: their brains are wired differently from ours. They get enjoyment from different experiences than we do, and many of the things we enjoy are stressful for them. It's up to us to love and appreciate them for their unique qualities—not to pressure them to our way of being. Doing that will only strain our relationship with them. It's our job to help them learn to appreciate and embrace their unique qualities.

The Low Ex Parent with a High Ex Child

Whereas High Ex parents with Low Ex children tend to *worry*, Low Ex parents with High Ex children tend to feel *guilty*. They feel like they can't keep up with their child; they feel like they should be giving their child more. You may love the enthusiasm with which your High Ex child experiences the world, but it can be so exhausting! Just reading about all the activities your High Ex child is likely to enjoy and ways to provide them social stimulation may feel overwhelming.

Don't despair! It *is* possible to find activities that will work for both of you; it just may require a bit more trial and error. As an extravert, your child is likely to want social stimulation; as an introvert, you may gravitate towards quieter activities. The ways you may have envisioned spending time with your child—reading a book together, doing puzzles, playing Go Fish—may not be sufficiently stimulating for them. That's not to say they won't want to do it at all (though if they are also low on Effortful Control, it might be challenging; more on that in chapter 6), but if you find them getting bored or frustrated, you know you need to mix in more of the social activities that your High Ex child craves.

This does not mean that you suddenly have to join the neighbourhood playgroup or spend your Saturday mornings making small talk with other parents on the playground (cringe). Try taking your High Ex child to activities where they can be around other children and get their fix of social interaction, but that are not too overwhelming for you. Believe it or not, there are outlets that will check both boxes. For example, you might see if your local library has a storytelling hour for children. Your High Ex child can be around other children, but you won't be forced to make small talk with a bunch of parents you don't know (or care to know). One of my Low Ex friends with a High Ex child found an educational hour at a local nature centre where an adult led a class about a different animal each week for the group of children; she would read quietly in the back of the room. Try working in playdates with a close friend, so it's not unbearable for you but your child gets the chance to develop their social skills. Look for opportunities like sports practices, or group activities like Scouting, where you can drop off your child. They get social interaction, and you get your much-needed quiet time. Look for after-school activities where they can be with other children and you can have some time to yourself. Importantly: *do not feel bad about this!* If you are constantly trying to be "on" for your child to keep them engaged, active, and happy, it will take a toll on you. Good parenting isn't about doing everything for your child; it's about figuring out what works best for you *and* your child. When parents and children are each in their own element, it makes everyone happier. And a happier parent is a better parent. So enjoy that after-school time alone!

Another thing that might not come naturally to you as a Low Ex parent is your High Ex child's need for feedback and approval. High Ex children are used to hearing things—whether it's their own voice or yours. They may interpret your lack of feedback as an indication that you aren't proud of them or that you disapprove. It will likely require effort on your part, but try to find ways to give them positive feedback. "Wow, you did a great job with that puzzle!" "You made so many new friends at the park today!" "You climbed so high on that tree!" High Ex children are often craving feedback from their quieter parents.

Finally, talk to your child about your different temperaments. Explain to them that you need quiet time on your own to recharge. Parents need their own space, and it's OK to tell your child that. You will be doing them a service by helping them understand that everyone's brains are wired differently, that some people need more quiet time to feel reenergised—and that you are one of those people. It is important to find a balance with your child from early on or else over time you may start to resent your High Ex child because it feels like they always want more from you—more talking, more activities, and more time with you.

Mismatched Siblings

If you have more than one child, chances are that they may differ in their level of Extraversion. This creates an extra challenge for parents. There is the logistical challenge of balancing your High Ex child's need for social activity with your Low Ex child's need for quiet time. But there is also the added challenge that your High Ex child may command more of your time and attention, making your Low Ex child feel overlooked and less valued compared to their more extraverted sibling.

The key to navigating family dynamics is to talk about it. Just as you may need to talk with your child about differences between your temperaments, you can use the differences between your children as an opportunity to teach them about how we all differ in our wiring for

Extraversion. Talk to your children about each of their unique strengths, so they understand how they are different, but both feel appreciated and valued. You can work with them to develop a team approach for how you are going to navigate their unique needs. Brainstorm and come up with plans together as a family. For example, if your High Ex child wants to go to a crowded museum and your Low Ex child protests, you can say, "What if we do the museum in the morning, and then Nathan gets to pick an activity for the afternoon?" Help your Low Ex child with ways they can take a break if the museum becomes too overwhelming—for example, by reading a book on a bench. If you find that your High Ex child is dominating dinner conversation, make it a point to ask your Low Ex child for their opinions. Encourage your High Ex child to let their Low Ex sibling speak. This will teach them to respect and value differences, which will serve them well in the long run. In short, it may present challenges and require some extra preparation, but having siblings who differ on Extraversion also offers a wonderful way to teach your children empathy and compromise.

Putting It All Together

Where our children naturally fall on Extraversion has a large impact on the way they experience and interact with the world. How we respond to their extraverted tendencies can create the scaffolding for that experience. One of the greatest gifts we can give our children is to help them understand and appreciate their unique strengths. Does our High Ex child feel loved for their high energy and enthusiasm, or resented because they are exhausting? Does our Low Ex child feel recognised for their quiet, creative, thoughtful character, or are they made to feel like they should be "more"? As parents, we can play a central role in how our children view their disposition. Both High Ex and Low Ex children have much to offer to the world, and it's up to us to help them discover that.

"Extroverts are fireworks, introverts are a fire in the hearth."
—Sophia Dembling

Takeaways

- Children show natural preferences at a young age for being around other people, and how much they like boisterous versus quiet activities. Many parenting stressors arise from mismatches between our child's natural temperament and the environments that we create for our children.

- High Ex children enjoy meeting new people, going new places, and trying new things. They are energised by being around others and quick to make friends, but they can also be exhausting, especially for parents who are not equally high on Extraversion.

- Low Ex children enjoy quiet activities and time alone or in smaller groups. Too much social stimulation can be overwhelming for them.

- High and Low Ex children need different things from their parents.

- High Ex children benefit from (1) feedback, (2) lots of social stimulation, (3) learning to slow down, and (4) learning to reflect and empathise.

- Low Ex children need (1) extra help to feel loved and accepted, (2) activities that fit their quieter disposition, (3) a quiet place of their own, and (4) help recognising when they need to take a break.

- Medium Ex children show some characteristics typical of High Ex children and some characteristics typical of Low Ex children. They are likely to enjoy a mixture of activities.

- Understanding what situations are likely to be a challenge for your child's temperament will help you to anticipate and prepare for them.

- When a child's level of Extraversion differs from their parents', it can cause stress and worry. Recognising these differences will help you navigate them. Siblings who differ in Extraversion also pose additional challenges.

- You can help your child understand the great things that come along with their particular temperament and teach them skills and strategies for the parts that are likely to pose challenges.

CHAPTER 5

· · · ▭ · · ·

Emotionality:
The "Em" Factor

When my son was at nursery, I'd plan an outing for us each Saturday morning—the park, the zoo, the children's museum—all the places I imagined us spending quality time together. On half these occasions we never even made it out the door. He'd be pulling on his shoes one minute, and in the next hurling those shoes through the air, then stomping to his room and slamming the door. What. Just. Happened?

As we discussed in chapter 3, children with high Emotionality are naturally prone to distress, frustration, and fear. My son is definitely High Em. If you have a High Em child, you know the territory: Outbursts that seem to come out of nowhere, complete freak-outs over . . . what? The most minor things. One minute you're happily colouring together, and the next they've torn their picture to pieces and stormed out of the room.

If you, too, are high Emotionality, you may well understand where the behaviour comes from, because you remember your own feelings as a child. You realise that the blue crayon must not have been the shade they were imagining for the sky, so the picture was "ruined!" But if you're low Emotionality, your child's behaviour may leave you completely baffled, probably even a little frightened.

If you have a Low Em child, you may be reading about outbursts and tantrums and wondering what the heck is wrong with these children . . . or with their parents. Misunderstandings about the genetics behind Emotionality lead to a lot of blame. Children who are high on Emotionality are called defiant, manipulative, attention-seeking, bratty, or spoiled. Parents with High Em children are judged for their child's emotional outbursts. They are described as too permissive, and poor disciplinarians. Other people may be quick to comment on their parenting—either directly, or to others: "They really need to teach that child to behave!"

Why are we so quick to blame parents for their children's behaviour? My girlfriends don't blame me when my husband does something ridiculous; they give me the knowing look of empathy. But that's not how we respond when it comes to other people's children. I think this is because for children lower on Emotionality, the standard toolbox of parenting strategies—redirecting, setting boundaries, consistent use of rewards and consequences—is pretty effective at shaping children's behaviour and minimising future misbehaviour (when implemented properly, which we'll get to). That's why parents of Low Em children look at parents with High Em children and think that those parents must be doing something wrong. Reward good behaviour, implement consequences for bad behaviour, and children learn to behave. Throwing shoes across the room earns a time-out; child learns not to throw shoes. It's the mainstream, commonsense view of proper parenting. Following that logic, if a child is consistently misbehaving, then it must be the parent who is doing something wrong. If only the parent implemented proper consequences, that child would learn to behave. Simple, right?

Not so fast. Children who are high on Emotionality, by definition, are unable to manage distress. So normal parental attempts to implement consequences when they are misbehaving simply escalates their distress. Contrary to popular belief, High Em children actually get *more* punishment and consequences, not less. If it appears that a fellow parent is being permissive with their child's misbehaviour in public, it's likely because that parent has learned that implementing consequences will only escalate the behaviour, and they are trying to spare everyone a scene. Unfortunately, that also perpetuates the idea that the behaviour results from permissive parenting and failure to implement consequences.

All of this blame and misunderstanding has at its roots the fact that children vary tremendously in their natural inclination towards Emotionality, and, importantly, different parenting strategies are needed for High versus Low Em children.

Because Emotionality is closely related to children's acting out, in this chapter we're going to cover effective strategies for shaping children's behaviour—that is, curbing tantrums *and* promoting desirable behaviour. We'll talk about which of these strategies work best for children with different levels of Emotionality. And I'll provide some additional suggestions for navigating family life with a High Em child.

The Perils of Punishment

We generally assume that there are some basic parenting principles that should work for all children. And the go-to parenting practice for dealing with disobedience is generally: punish bad behaviour. Think for a second about how ingrained into our psyche that principle is: Children need to learn to respect authority. They need to understand who is in charge. They need to know who's boss. Children need to learn the consequences of their actions (and generally, as parents, we interpret that to mean that *we* need to implement consequences). Spare the rod, spoil the child. We think it's our duty to teach them the way the world works: when you do bad things, bad things follow.

This is how many of us were raised. It's what comes naturally to many parents. Child misbehaves, parent punishes. It feels so intuitive that we don't even stop to ask where the idea came from. You may be surprised to learn that this common parenting practice dates back to the time when men were legally responsible for their wives, children, and animals. If women or children acted up, the husband/father was held legally responsible; accordingly, men were allowed to do "whatever it took" to keep their women and children in line. Tragically, this widely accepted view led to the abuse of many women and children. As a culture, our views on relationships between men and women, and on the treatment of women, have evolved substantially. We no longer accept the once widely held practice of husbands hitting their wives to get them to "behave". While our views on corporal punishment of children have also evolved over the years, the general idea that bad behaviour should be punished continues to be mainstream. As a friend once said to me, "There's nothing like some good old-fashioned parenting to keep kids in line".

I'm going to ask you to be open-minded for a minute, and try to imagine a different way of parenting children. Our historical tendencies towards stern parenting are so ingrained that a softer approach may feel foreign, or too touchy-feely. But just for a minute, let's suspend our preconceived ideas and turn to the science behind what works to shape children's behaviour. Because most of us would like to have well-behaved children. Or realistically, at least better-behaved children.

Here's what the research shows: punishment doesn't work. Sure, it might stop the behaviour in the moment. But contrary to what most parents think, *it doesn't change the likelihood that the behaviour will occur again in the future.* That's because punishment doesn't teach our children what we want them to do. Instead, it teaches them behaviour we don't want them to display. When we shout, it teaches them that when they are cross about something, they shout. Hitting teaches hitting. What children learn from punishment is that if you want to get your way, if you want to impose your will on someone, if you don't like what someone is doing, you shout, hit, or punish them. That probably isn't the lesson you were intending to convey.

The other irony is that punishment actually focuses attention on behaviours we don't want kids to repeat. Parental attention is a form of reward for children. So when we gripe and nag about bad behaviour, we are rewarding the behaviours we don't like. Too often, when children are doing what they are supposed to be doing, we don't say anything. We quietly and peaceably go about the day and enjoy those blissful moments of calm. But that means we are actually ignoring the behaviour we want to see more of. Children quickly learn that if they want mum or dad's attention, they are far more likely to get it by taunting their sibling than by colouring nicely. Eating dinner properly goes without mention, but spitting milk through their nose definitely gets a response! Too often we fail to acknowledge good behaviour, but bad behaviour gets a rise out of parents with regularity.

Parents will frequently ask: but isn't punishing a way for children to learn right from wrong? Spoiler alert: your child already knows right from wrong. Your child isn't failing to brush their teeth because they don't know they are supposed to brush. They aren't hitting their sibling because they didn't know they weren't supposed to hit. I'm willing to bet you've told them plenty of times to brush their teeth, or to not hit their sibling. Both Low Em and High Em children are very good at describing what they should or should not be doing when they are not in the middle of mischief. They can tell you what behaviour is OK and not OK, why it's wrong, and they can tell you what will happen if they do it. *But that still doesn't stop them from doing it.*

Part of the reason that punishment doesn't work is that simply knowing something is wrong doesn't automatically stop the behaviour in the future. I know that eating an entire carton of ice cream is not a good idea. That alone doesn't stop me. I know that I should exercise more; that alone does not inspire me to jump out of bed each morning at six a.m. and pull on my running shoes.

The final problem with punishment is that kids quickly adapt to it. This means that in order for punishment to have the desired effect of stopping misbehaviour, you have to keep upping the ante. Anyone who has ever lost it with a toddler has seen this—the first time you raise your voice, it startles them; over time the shock value wears off. This means that you have to keep escalating the punishment to get a response—shout louder, lecture longer—or in the days when smacking was more widely used—hit harder. Obviously, this starts a cycle that isn't good for anyone. It doesn't stop the behaviour in the moment. It requires you to escalate to more and more severe punishment (and where does that end?). It doesn't decrease the frequency of the behaviour in the future. Losing your temper doesn't make you feel good as a parent. And it's probably hurting your relationship with your child. So why is punishment our go-to technique as parents? Turns out it's just a pretty ineffective historical relic. Kind of like keeping women in their place. We're long overdue for some new strategies with our children.

The alternative to punishing bad behaviour is to work on promoting good behaviour. It's actually much easier to build up good behaviour than to get rid of bad behaviour. And the more time kids spend being good, the less time they spend being bad. It's like magic! It has been called *positive parenting*, and you've probably come across it in a parenting blog or book. There's heaps of research showing that it's good for children, and we're going to walk through the scientifically backed strategies that work. But there's one more key piece: there are slightly different strategies that are more effective for Low and High Em children. If you have a High Em child, you may find that the standard toolbox is not enough. Don't worry: there's a whole section with extra strategies for you.

Just like training a puppy, building good behaviour starts by rewarding it. The most powerful tool we have as parents is not punishment, but reward. Rewarding good behaviour reinforces the behaviour you want to see more of. It calls attention to good behaviour, rather than focusing on the bad. And it's far more fun to do as a parent. But for it to work, you have to do it right.

Rewarding the Right Way

All rewards are not created equal, and by that, I don't mean that an iPhone is more desirable than an ice cream. The way you implement rewards can have a big impact on whether they alter your child's behaviour. It's not uncommon for parents to come into the clinic and say that they tried rewarding, but it didn't work. Rewarding only works to shape child behaviour when it is implemented properly. Here are the basic principles of how to implement rewards in a way that will actually change child behaviour.

Pay attention to good behaviour. The first pillar of increasing good behaviour effectively is to pay attention to good behaviour. That may sound silly, but think about how often we say nothing when our child is going about their business doing the things they are supposed to be doing. We ask them to brush their teeth. Put on their pajamas. Get in the bath. Get in bed. And when they do it, very frequently we say nothing. We simply expect them to do what they are supposed to, and we all go about our day. It's when they splash an entire bathtub's worth of water on the floor that they get a reaction. When they are playing with their toys instead of putting on pajamas that we start to gripe. When they are jumping on the new sofa, or tracking mud across the kitchen floor, that's when mums and dads come running.

So how do we change the cycle? Instead of catching our kids being bad, we have to focus on recognising the positive behaviour. The keys to rewarding properly (i.e. in a way that will result in the desired behaviour increasing in the future) are to be (1) enthusiastic, (2) specific, (3) immediate, and (4) consistent.

Start by attending to and enthusiastically commenting on good behaviour. Don't just comment in passing; channel your inner cheerleader to summon a degree of enthusiasm about putting on underwear that you never dreamed possible before you had children. "What a great job you did putting on your underwear!" Be specific and name the good behaviour, rather than speaking in generalities. In other words, don't just say "Good job!" or "You're being so good," say "Great job brushing your teeth!" "Nice job putting on your pajamas!" "Wow, you got dressed so quickly today!" "Look at you eating cereal with your spoon!"

You need to reward the good behaviour immediately when it occurs, and every time that it occurs. If your child is having trouble getting dressed in a timely manner, then comment on what a great job they did getting dressed *as soon as they are dressed*, not later that day when you are running errands. And do it every morning until the good behaviour is established. "Yay, you put on your underwear again today!"

How easily verbally rewarding your child comes to you is likely a product of your own upbringing and personality. I grew up in a family with lots of positive praise, and now I'm a psychologist. So there is a lot of positive feedback in our house. It makes my husband laugh that even as adults when we see my parents, I can mention the smallest accomplishment ("I paid bills today") and my parents respond with effuse praise ("That's great that you got your bills done! Doesn't it feel good!"). He thinks it's funny. But it *does* feel good, and that positive feedback even makes paying bills seem a little more enjoyable.

If this all feels a bit silly to you, think of it this way: you are the boss of your child (despite how frequently they tell you you're not). What kind of boss would you want to work for? Probably a boss who notices when you are doing what you're supposed to be doing, who points out and celebrates your accomplishments. No one wants to work for a boss who jumps on them every time they do something wrong, who never mentions all the times they are doing something right. People like bosses who are warm, understanding, and supportive; bosses who realise that sometimes people make mistakes, but they allow you to learn from those mistakes and they don't dwell on them. Research shows that people who work for bosses with these qualities are happier and more productive. This is true of our children too.

Take baby steps. That's all fine and good, you may be thinking, but the problem is that my child *doesn't* put on their clothes, so I have nothing to reward. The key here is to start small. Start by rewarding steps in the right direction, and gradually build from there. If your child is currently refusing to get dressed in the morning, you could start by rewarding them for simply picking out their clothes. Or you could reward them for pulling on underwear only. If the problem is the amount of time it takes them to get dressed, you could set it up as a "beat the clock" race. Start by being generous. If it usually takes thirty minutes, give them twenty minutes. Then cut back to fifteen, then to ten. Baby steps. Once your child starts to recognise that rewards follow from doing what they are asked, they will be willing to do more and more. The key is to break it down into small, manageable steps.

It's also important to reward each behaviour individually. You don't want to collapse several behaviours together for your child to earn a reward. For example, you don't want to try to reward "a smoother evening routine". You want to break that down into the components of the evening routine (brush teeth, put on pajamas, get in bed) and then work on, and reward, the individual behaviours that make up the routine.

Focus on what matters. You don't need to reward your child's every behaviour. Focus on the behaviours that are creating challenges at home. Depending on the child, there may be a few . . . or many. The reality is that you can't work on everything at once. Pick a few areas that you are going to focus on changing through a conscious reward system (I recommend no more than three at a time). Think back to the type of boss you would want to work for: if they gave you a list of twenty things that need improvement immediately, you would likely feel overwhelmed and none of them would happen. If they gave you two or three, you could work on those, get them accomplished, feel good about it, and once they became routine, you would be encouraged and ready to move on to the next items. The same is true of our children. You can only focus on a few behaviours at once or else everyone loses track. I have seen sticker charts so elaborate that you need a Ph.D. to follow them.

If you're only working on a few behaviours at a time, what are you supposed to do when other bad behaviour occurs? Ignore it. This is probably the hardest part for parents. *Ignore bad behaviour?!* I know it feels counter-intuitive, but it works. Remember that attention is a form of reward, so you don't want to inadvertently reward bad behaviour at the same time you're trying to focus on growing good behaviour. Prioritise the most important behaviours and ignore the rest (for the time being). So if you're working on the evening routine, and they are still slurping milk out of their cereal bowl—ignore it. Ignoring means no verbal, physical, or eye contact. If you have to, leave the room.

Obviously you can't ignore things like hitting or throwing things, or not following your directions. But a lot of the annoying things kids do we can ignore, including whining, throwing tantrums, pouting, showing off, badgering you for attention. The key is that once you start ignoring, you have to keep ignoring. This is likely to escalate the behaviour—your child will try even harder to get your attention. If you give in, you've just re-warded ramping up the bad behaviour. So stay strong! This is a strategy for the long haul; over time it will decrease bad behaviour, I promise you. And when your child stops whining? Immediately reward the good be-haviour! "Thank you so much for sitting quietly while mum talks on the phone!" Never mind that they spent fifteen minutes whining at you and are only sitting quietly because they wore themselves out; don't mention that. As soon as they are sitting quietly, immediately praise that behaviour and pretend the other never happened. It's a skill to be cultivated.

Use rewards to stop bad behaviour. How do you focus on rewards when what you really want is for your child to *stop* doing something? Dawdling in the morning, picking on their sibling, leaving dirty clothes strewn about—there are arrays of frustrating child behaviours that we parents would like to put an end to. There's a way to use rewards for that too. Dr Alan Kazdin, a child psychologist at Yale who has done extensive work with families, calls it "focusing on the positive oppo-site". In other words, rather than calling attention to the behaviour you want your child to stop, focus instead on what you want them to do—the positive opposite of the problematic behaviour. So instead of trying to stop the dawdling or the squabbling, instead focus on rewarding your child when they do what they are supposed to—pulling on their clothes in the morning in a timely manner, a dinner that passes without a sibling argument, a bedroom floor that does not have yesterday's socks lying about. When that happens, those are behaviours worth rewarding; over time you can replace the annoying behaviour with its positive opposite.

Using the Right Reward

So far we've focused on verbal rewards: praising your child. Don't underestimate the power of verbal rewards. Effusive, warm praise from a parent, accompanied by hugs and cuddles, can be a powerful reward for children. Remember: channel your inner cheerleader!

But for more challenging or stubborn behaviours, you may need a more salient reward system. This is where reward charts come in, where the immediate reward is putting a sticker (or a tick mark) on a chart to work towards a larger or a later reward. Anything your child enjoys can be used as a reward: a trip to a favourite park, playing a favourite game together, getting a special treat. You can work with your child to create a reward "bank" of things they are excited to work towards. When kids participate in the process, they are more likely to be excited about it. You can even do a "trial run" to jump-start the connection between good behaviour and rewards. For example, if the behaviour you are working on is teeth brushing, and you decide that the reward will be putting a sticker on the chart, where three stickers earn a special treat, then you can say, "Let's practise! Go pretend like you're brushing your teeth, and then we'll put a sticker on the chart!" Assuming they comply (even if it's begrudgingly or involves lacklustre brushing), then you immediately put a sticker on the chart and say, "Look! You already have one sticker! You only need two more to get your treat!"

If your child refuses to participate in a trial run, you just calmly say, "OK, we can try again later when you're ready". No lecturing, no nagging. In my experience, when enough time had passed that my son felt like it was "his" idea and not mine, nine times out of ten he would declare, "I'm going to brush my teeth now". When your child finally relents in this way and does the task, respond with effuse praise (even if you are frustrated). Don't point out that they could have received the sticker an hour ago. Or sarcastically say that you're glad they've come around. Imagine if you announced that you were going to tackle the laundry and your partner said, "You mean the laundry you said you were going to do last week?" That would not inspire you to run to the laundry room faster. In fact, it would probably turn your mood to grumpy and make you less likely to do the laundry. Remember, you only want positive associations with the good behaviour you want to grow. "Great! Nice job teeth brushing!" It's the parent equivalent of, "Thanks so much for doing the laundry, honey!" and biting one's tongue when it comes to any other editorialising.

If you do use reward charts, remember to always accompany a sticker reward with praise, to keep it simple, and to be generous with your rewards. A child who has to collect ten stickers to get a reward may get bored with the system before the reward kicks in. Remember that you want to have the opportunity to start connecting good behaviour with rewards. If your child is getting frustrated with how long or hard it is to get their reward, you are defeating the purpose. There's no need to be mean with rewards.

I've also had parents ask me if children are more likely to get excited about reward charts if they are more "fun", i.e. they have pictures of their favourite superhero or are brightly coloured. If you want to make a fabulous, impressive star chart to post on Pinterest, more power to you. And certainly, working with your child to create a chart together can be a fun bonding activity. But there is no evidence that children comply any more readily with a fabulous *Frozen* reward chart than a few lines drawn on a piece of paper. So if art isn't your thing, don't sweat it. As long as you are doing the key pieces (rewarding enthusiastically, immediately, and consistently, and working on specific, small steps), that's all that matters.

Phasing Out

You may find yourself wondering if you will be making sticker charts forever. The good news is that once our brains make a connection between behaviour and reward, you can gradually phase out the reward and the behaviour will continue. You may have received rewards for using the toilet as a small child. Presumably you are not still expecting M&Ms every time you go to the loo. I promise you will not be giving stars for teeth brushing to your sixth former (unless maybe you have a boy; I'm not sure they ever internalise regular hygiene).

How long, you ask, will it take to establish the connection before you can phase out the reward? That will depend on your child. For most children, it takes a few weeks to a couple months. Once the behaviour is occurring regularly and feels like it is a normal part of the routine, then you're probably ready to move on to the next behaviour you want to work on. It's still a good idea to keep giving verbal praise. And if there is a regression when you move on to the next behaviour, you know you stopped too soon. It wasn't ingrained yet. No problem: just revert back to your system and keep on a bit longer.

Why Should I Reward My Child for Things They Should Already Be Doing? And Other Common Concerns

The most common complaint I hear from parents is: why should I reward my child for things they should be doing anyway? The reality is that there are lots of things we all should be doing. I should go to the gym more often. I should eat healthier. I should make the bed. Yes, your child should tidy their room right away when you ask, but they're no more likely to do that than you are to stick to that six a.m. body-sculpting class you promised yourself you'd start attending daily in the new year. You can wax poetic about what your child should be doing, and you can keep getting frustrated at them for not doing it. Or you can use science to help shape their behaviour.

Another common parent concern that gets raised: isn't it a bad idea to bribe my child into doing the right thing? To be clear, rewards aren't bribes. Bribes are payments used to get someone to do something they *shouldn't* be doing. You're trying to increase behaviour the child *should* be doing. We all work for rewards. We go to work because we get paid. We do the body-sculpting class because we feel healthier afterwards (and maybe start to lose a few extra pounds). I am more likely to make the bed when my husband tells me how much he appreciates it.

Remember, human brains are wired for reward. The things we find rewarding, we continue to do, and we do them more often. By rewarding your child for the behaviour you want them to display, you are simply using science to help your child learn good behaviour.

The Other Lever: Consequences

So now you're practising your superior parenting skills: attending to good behaviour; giving rewards that are enthusiastic, specific, immediate, and consistent; rewarding small, individual behaviours (or steps to work up to the full behaviour); and ignoring other bad behaviour that is not the current priority. Your child is now perfect, right? If only. Inevitably your child will do something you can't ignore: they will hit their sibling, they will look at you defiantly and scoot their dinner plate off the table, they will throw the bath toy at you when you tell them it is time to get out of the bath. These are things you can't ignore. So now we get to the part that so many parents seem to know best: consequences.

Once you are into the routine of rewarding good behaviour, you will have to use consequences far less frequently. But you will still have to use them. Just like rewards, there's a right way to give consequences to make them effective. First, don't instruct your child to do something unless you are willing to follow through on it—meaning, if they don't comply, there will be a consequence. If it's not that big a deal to you, or you're not in a position to implement a consequence (either you're busy with something else or in a public place where you really don't want to get into it), then practise your ignoring skill. But once you have issued a directive, if your child doesn't comply, then you have to implement a consequence. Otherwise, what you've taught your child is that they don't have to listen to you all of the time.

Remember that it's always better to issue a positive directive than a negative one. Say "Keep your hands in the cart" when you are shopping, rather than "Don't pull things off the shelves". Focus on the positive opposite—the behaviour you want to see rather than the behaviour you don't want to see. (Note: This takes a while to get used to, but once you're in the rhythm, I promise it starts to come naturally.) Many times there are obvious natural consequences you can use. For example, if the child swipes some cereal boxes off the shelf, their consequence can be picking them up and putting them back nicely.

Consequences Done Right

Just as with rewards, for consequences to work—meaning that they will help reduce the behaviour in the future—you have to implement them *immediately* and *consistently*. Time-outs are a go-to consequence favourite because they can be implemented virtually anywhere, whether you're at home or in the supermarket. Time-outs essentially consist of the removal of positive rewards, i.e. no contact with you, or other things the child finds rewarding. A good rule of thumb is usually about a minute per the child's age, so three minutes in time-out for a three-year-old. Many parents have a time-out chair at home, or use a corner at the shop if needed. Several of the parenting books included in the Resources and Recommended Readings section at the end of this book (*1-2-3 Magic, The Kazdin Method*, and *Parenting the Strong-Willed Child*) have additional information about implementing time-outs effectively. But for most children, any variation that removes positive rewards (including your attention) will work. The key piece is to implement a consequence *every time* the child fails to follow your direction.

Another surprising fact about consequences is that the gravity of the consequence does not affect how well it works to decrease that behaviour in the future. In other words, removing a favourite toy for a week is no more effective than losing the toy for the remainder of the day. The most effective consequences are mild, immediate, and brief. Parents, I know you hate this. I certainly do. It feels like the punishment doesn't fit the crime. But the most critical piece for a consequence to work is having a consequence in the first place. In fact, bigger consequences may actually be counter-effective because they give the child lots of time to build up resentment towards you, and they remove its immediacy. When their bike gets taken away for a week, and they ask to ride it several days into the week and you say no, the reason that the bike was taken away is now days away, so it feels like you are just being mean. The direct connection between the bad behaviour and the consequence has been lost.

Here are a few last things to consider about consequences. First, you never want to have a consequence be a behaviour that you want the child to do anyway. For example, don't assign raking leaves as a consequence if you want the child to help out with gardening generally. Don't assign doing the washing up if you are trying to instill helping around the house as a good behaviour that is expected.

Finally, and perhaps most importantly, don't instill consequences when you are angry. Yes, I left the hardest piece for last. The reality is that the behaviours that merit consequences are also likely to upset us (Did you really just talk to me that way?!). When we are angry, it ramps up our desire to dole out consequences. But it's also the time that we are most likely to use consequences ineffectively. I remember taking my son bowling when he was younger, with the idea that it would be a fun bonding afternoon together. It ended with him throwing a massive fit when I wouldn't move to a lane with gutter bumpers partway through the game and me shouting, "I will never take you bowling again, *ever*!" A good example of why not to dole out consequences when you're angry.

The Parenting Tool Kit Summarised— and When It Falls Short

The table below pulls together everything we've learned so far about how to use rewards and consequences effectively to shape child behaviour. If you have a child who is low to medium on Emotionality, it's a scientifically backed, tried-and-true tool kit that will make a big difference if you implement it consistently.

EFFECTIVELY SHAPING CHILD BEHAVIOUR
Attend to good behaviour
Ignore bad behaviour
Focus on a small number of behaviours at a time
Reward small steps
Rewards should be: • Enthusiastic—think cheerleader • Specific—name the good behaviour • Immediate—reward when the behaviour occurs • Consistent—reward the behaviour every time it occurs
Consequences should be: • Used only when you can't ignore • Immediate and consistent • Less is more—will almost never "fit the crime" • Only implemented when you are calm

But if you have a High Em child, you may find that the standard parenting strategies of implementing rewards and consequences isn't working. In fact, it may be making the behaviour *worse*. When parents with High Em kids start reward and consequence programmes, often their children spend inordinate amounts of time in time-out (or experiencing other consequences), and rarely earn rewards. High Em children may start to internalise the idea that they are "bad" because there is now a system in place that documents how much they are failing their parents' expectations. Parents become increasingly despondent that things are never going to get better. They wonder what they are doing wrong (or come down hard on what the *other* is doing wrong), or they fear that there may be something wrong with their child. In short, everybody is upset, the behaviour isn't getting better, and your relationship with your child is getting worse. What's going on?

Rewards and consequences work by helping children make connections between the behaviour you want to see (and conversely, don't want to see), and giving them an incentive to behave accordingly. When High Em children continue to misbehave, we tend to conclude they just need more incentive to stop misbehaving, hence the doubling down on consequences. But High Em children aren't lacking the *motivation* to behave properly, they are lacking the *skills*. They were born with a disposition towards strong emotions, towards distress and frustration. They can't naturally manage these emotions. If you had a child struggling to read, or to do algebra, you wouldn't expect that rewards and consequences would teach them their ABCs, or the Pythagorean theorem. Punishing them for their inability to read or do algebra is actually cruel, and would likely cause your child to start to resent you.

That's what happens when High Em children are constantly being punished for their behaviour. Parents become a target of their High Em child's frustration and anger, which further angers parents. In chapter 2, we talked about how our genotypes influence the way other people respond to us. High Em children evoke negative reactions from their parents. Their High Em genotypes are really good at triggering our wrath, and then it's off to the races in a feedback loop that escalates everyone's bad behaviour and leads to nothing but further anger and frustration. You ask them to do something, they refuse, you double down on your demand, perhaps accompanied by a consequence ("You're going to lose your favourite toy if you don't stop kicking the back of the seat!"), they ramp up the bad behaviour to let you know how much they don't appreciate the threat, and the next thing you know, everyone's cross.

My dear friend tells the story of how her High Em child's refusal to stop tapping her fork on the dinner table culminated in her husband emerging from their daughter's bedroom drowning under an armful of princess dresses and stuffed animals. Apparently, in the heat of one final fork bang before a huffy departure to her room, my friend's husband yelled after their daughter, "If you don't come back and politely finish dinner, you are going to lose your pink princess dress!" To which his smart High Em child replied, "No problem, I have lots more", which led to the removal of stuffed animals too, just for good measure!

If you've had a version of this scene play out at your house, don't despair. You haven't been sentenced to eighteen years of tantrums and talking back, you just need some additional tools in your toolbox. That's what we'll cover next.

Parenting Strategies for High Em Children (With More Tips for Low Em Kids Too!)

All children have challenges, and if you have more than one child, in all likelihood each one will struggle in a different way. The first step to helping your High Em child is to *remember that he or she didn't ask to be this way*, any more than she or he asked to have a reading disability or maths anxiety. It's not a choice. It's coded in their genes. The minute you accept that and begin to see the situation through that lens, the easier life becomes.

The second step is to remember that what High Em kids need—the kids who are often the holy terrors who can drive you to your own limits—is *not a firmer hand* but warmer and gentler discipline. This is sometimes hard to accept, because it's exactly the opposite of most parents' natural inclination, which is to come down hard on behaviour that seems completely out of line.

It makes you crazy when your child crumples the art project that they have been working on all afternoon. And when the outburst happens in public, with seemingly the whole world watching and disapproving, the pressure mounts to *do something about that unacceptable behaviour.*

But again, this kind of cracking down only creates a negative feed-back loop. The child gets angrier, which makes the parent more upset, which makes the child get more worked up, and on and on.

As the parent of a High Em child, you need to help them learn to manage their strong feelings. The first step is shifting focus away from the *behaviour* and towards the *triggers* of this temperamental tendency. That alone can start to short-circuit the negative feedback loop. Ideally, you'll then be able to help your child channel all that emotional energy into more suitable outlets.

You've identified that you have a High Em child, which means that the "bad" behaviour—sudden outbursts, temper tantrums—is often a by-product, a signal, and not really where the action is. Your High Em kiddo is simply more sensitive to their environment, expects more from it, from themselves, and from you! That's a lot for a little brain to handle.

As I said at the outset, I may be an expert in behavioural develop-ment, but I'm also a mum, and for me it took a while to get beyond the natural tendency to simply snap back when snapped at. Before I could fully appreciate what was going on and allow myself to transfer what I knew intellectually into daily practice, Saturday mornings with my son went something like this:

ME: "Guess what? We're going to get together with Jake and Madeline and Sara and Paul and their mummies and daddies and all go to the playground! It's going to be so much fun! Pull on your shoes, and let's head out!"

MY HIGH EM CHILD: "I don't want to go."

ME: "Of course you want to go; come on, it'll be fun."

MY HIGH EM CHILD: "No, I don't want to go."

ME: "Well, we're going, so pull on your shoes."

MY HIGH EM CHILD: "I'm not going."

ME: "Yes, you are; you don't get to make the rules. I've already told everyone we'll be there. Now come on, we're going to be late."

MY HIGH EM CHILD: "I'M. NOT. GOING." *(Throws shoes at me.)*

ME: "That is absolutely unacceptable. You do not throw things! Go to time-out."

MY HIGH EM CHILD: "No." *(Sits down on floor and refuses to move.)*

ME *(Raising Voice)*: "I said Go. To. Time-out."

MY HIGH EM CHILD: *"No!"*

You don't have to be an "expert" to see that this is going nowhere good. It's certainly not leading to a fun day at the park with friends.

After I did a little more thinking, aligning my observations of my son with the basics of what I knew about genetic predispositions, I realised what was contributing to the Saturday morning meltdowns. After reading the last chapter, you can probably recognise the root of the problem now too. As I have shared, my son is low on Extraversion. In contrast, I'm the consummate people-person. That was creating a mismatch. In my world, fun meant being around all my friends and having our children play together on the slides and swings.

But what sounded like the perfect day for me sounded like misery for my more introverted son. Springing on him the idea that we were headed out to a large gathering of people was more than he could handle. His toddler brain didn't have the maturity to say, "Mum, I feel anxious when I'm around so many people; do you think we could just do a quiet play-date with one close friend?" Instead, his distress impulse led him to panic, which activated his high Emotionality, and the shoe flying across the room was simply collateral damage.

How do you figure out your High Em child's triggers? The time to do this is *not* when your child is already upset. When your child is in distress, they experience a physiological reaction that blocks their ability to think clearly. And this mental "white out" doesn't happen only to children. Think about the last time that your partner did something to really tick you off. You probably were not at your best. Most likely you experienced increased heart rate, tension, and an inability to think logically and clearly—all physical reactions tied in to the "fight-or-flight" response.

Oddly enough, we often hold our children to a higher standard than we do ourselves. "Just calm down. It's really not a big deal; don't get so worked up." Imagine if your partner said, "What's the big deal?" to you when you were really upset about something. It probably wouldn't go down too well. In fact, the minimising is likely to make you even more upset. "How dare you invalidate my feelings! Don't tell me what's a big deal and what isn't! This *is* a big deal!"

It will be many years before your little one has an "executive brain" that's sufficiently developed to express strong feelings in a calm manner. (Let's be honest, it's even hard for those of us who do have fully developed brains!) So what does your child do to try to express the fear, anxiety, and frustration? They throw their shoe across the room, or trash their art project. The words simply aren't available to adequately express "I'm really upset!" Their strong feelings are just too much to handle.

Think about how you would want your partner to respond when you're worked up over something. Probably by listening to you, understanding where you're coming from, and trying to figure out how to make it better in the future. You want him or her to work with you, not to tell you all the reasons you're being ridiculous, or "childish", or how much he or she dislikes it when you get this way.

That's exactly what your High Em child needs as well. To be heard. To be comforted. To be loved for who they are. The best way to deal with High Em children is with compassion—to understand their feelings, and come up with a plan for how you are going to work together to handle challenging situations that are bound to arise in the future.

I've had parents say to me, "But you can't reason with a child!" That's true—in the moment when they're upset. Just as it's true that I don't want my husband to say to me, "Honey, let's talk about how we can more productively discuss our differences", when I'm really laying into him about the laundry that is *still* piled on the sofa a week after he said he would put it away.

When someone is upset—whether that someone is three or thirty-three—it's not a great time to have a productive conversation. But once your little one has settled down, you can have a conversation about what got them so worked up, and how to ward off showdowns in the future. It's only by understanding the *why* behind the High Em behaviour that you can help your child channel it towards something better. And there's no better way to figure out the *why* than by talking with your child.

Partners in Crime:
Building a Collaborative Relationship with Your High Em Child

Too often, high Emotionality leads parents and children into a pattern where they are set against each other. That's not enjoyable, or productive, for anyone. A central component to getting on the right track is to shift from being in a standoff with your High Em child to being on the same side. We're going to walk through a few simple steps you can follow to work with your child to help them manage their natural tendency towards strong emotions.

Discover your child's triggers. Part of what makes High Em children's behaviour so upsetting is that their fits seem to be "over nothing" or come "out of nowhere". The fact that your child *can* be a delightful little being (sometimes) perpetuates the idea that they are *choosing* not to behave. That mindset is what gets us into the cycle of imposing consequences—to try to motivate them to behave. But remember that High Em children are not choosing to get worked up. Something is *triggering* their disposition towards frustration, distress, or fear. Your job is to work with your child as a pair of detectives to figure out what those triggers are.

There are a number of common triggers for High Em children (see the following table). These include things like transitioning between activities, completing tasks that are challenging, changes in plans, and when things don't turn out as the child had hoped. All of the triggers are related to the High Em child's natural disposition towards higher levels of frustration, distress, and fear. The way your child's High Em disposition manifests will be specific to your child. Not all High Em children have trouble with all of these tasks (though some do). Look through this list as a starting place for decoding what's triggering your child's tantrums. Start a list of triggers for your High Em child, along with examples of specific problems your child is having. If none of the triggers jump out at you, keep a journal of times and situations when your child gets upset so you can begin to identify patterns and create your own list.

COMMON HIGH EM TRIGGERS	EXAMPLES
Change in plans	It's raining so you can't go to the park.
Completing tasks that are challenging	A class assignment that the child doesn't want to do.
When things don't turn out as hoped	A picture that didn't turn out as intended.
Transitioning between activities	Time to stop playing in the bath and put on pajamas.
When something/someone is not available	Their friend can't make a standing playdate.
Getting things done under pressure	It's time to leave for school in thirty minutes.
Managing ambiguity	We can only go to the playground if it doesn't rain tomorrow.
Sensory issues	The tag on their clothes "feels funny".
Anxiety	They are nervous about being in the school play.
Difficulty expressing feelings	Kicks a child.
Overwhelmed by too many people/activities	Gets upset when at a birthday party or large playdate.

With High Em kiddos, the key is to focus on *problem-solving*, rather than rewarding and punishing behaviour. Using rewards and consequences assumes that your child just needs incentives to behave in a certain way. Remember: the problem is not that High Em children are lacking motivation—they are lacking the ability to manage their strong emotions. Your child probably doesn't want to lose control and throw fits any more than you want them to. In fact, their inability to control their strong feelings probably scares them as much as it does you.

When my son was about five years old, he threw the mother of all fits at the doctor's office. He had a sore throat. I took him to the doctor and they needed to swab his throat to test for Streptococcal tonsillitis. Most children don't like having a long swab stuck down their throat. A Low Em child might protest, and may even cry. My High Em child dug in and refused to open his mouth.

First we coaxed and dangled a reward. "It will be super fast and then we can go for ice cream! It won't hurt a bit!" He didn't budge. We switched tactics. Stern voice: "I know you are afraid, but it's not a choice. We have to do the test." No change. So we switched again and moved on to consequences: "Young man, you are going to open your mouth right now or you will lose your Legos!" That got a response, but not the one we wanted. "No!" he yelled angrily, and kicked the doctor. I will spare you the details of what happened next, but it involved crawling under the table, pushing over chairs, and an entire team of nurses who eventually held him down to get the throat swab as he screamed at the top of his lungs. It was awful. When we got home, we both went to our respective bedrooms and cried.

Then, under my door, he slipped me a little note. I have kept it to this day. It is folded into a tiny booklet, written in kindergarten writing, and says:

> *To Mom. By Aidan. Dear Mom, I am scared about throwing a fit at the docter. I will try to never do it again. I am scared about throwing your phone. I will try never do it again. I am*

so so so so so so so sarea [sorry]! I was so mad because the docters were herting my hip so so much [we later discovered he had a rare hip disorder]. Now my hip is so so so sor. And I didn't want to get the long thing in my mouth cuse I alwase think about it getting stuck dawn my throte. So I do not like to do it. After they put the long thing in my mouth I had some cotin stuck in my throte. I am very saree [sorry]. Can you forgive me? A) yes B) no

I keep that note because it reminds me that this is not a child who was trying to misbehave. High Em children aren't just being defiant, or bratty, or trying to get their way. They actually have different wiring, a different genetic make-up. They are dealing with overwhelming emotions that they don't know how to manage. When we double down on consequences (or make fleeting abandoned attempts at rewards), we only make them feel worse about themselves. No one wins.

Oh, and in case you were wondering, the throat swab was negative.

Collaborate to problem-solve. Once you have your list of triggers, along with the specific examples of challenges your High Em child is having, it's time to start problem-solving. Choose a few of the problems that represent your biggest concerns to focus on first. This doesn't mean you will never get to the others; it just means that you have to start somewhere, and you can't tackle everything at once. Remember the boss you want to be—the one who gives you manageable chunks to work on at a time, not the one who overloads you with a long list of tasks that are all due immediately.

The key to successful problem-solving is that your child has to be an equal partner. You have likely already attempted a lot of problem-solving on your own. You have probably read parenting advice and implemented things like the standard rewards and consequences we discussed earlier. As parents, we feel responsible for coming up with solutions for our children's problems. We are the ones who are used to having the answers. So it may feel strange at first to work with your child to come up with solutions.

But when you come up with a plan on your own, you are imposing your ideas on your child. Although these plans are well-meaning, think about that for a minute: You are *imposing your ideas* on your *easily frustrated, highly emotional* child. Sadly, this means most parental attempts to make the problem better actually have the opposite effect. They create another trigger for their High Em child. You are perceived as being inflexible, and that doesn't help your child learn to be more flexible. Your High Em child is likely to respond with equally strong inflexibility, which just further perpetuates the negative cycle.

You can change that. Try to think of it as a relief—it's not all on your shoulders! You get to work with your child to figure out how to address their challenges. It gets to be a collaborative process that puts you and your child on the same team to work together to tackle their high Emotionality. Together you are going to come up with a plan. This enables you to shift from being reactive to proactive. Most families with a High Em child are in reactive mode—they are trying to do damage control when their child has an outburst. By figuring out your child's triggers, and working on their specific problems, you can proactively come up with a plan for how to manage those strong feelings when they get triggered.

This will not be a once-and-for-all conversation with your child. It will be a process. Pick a time to start the conversation when you and your child are both well rested, in a good mood, and you aren't pushed for time. Start with empathy. Remember that your child's High Em outbursts are probably as scary for them as they are for you. Give them space to talk about what is going on, and to understand your child's perspective on what is triggering them. Just like with my son's note, when High Em children are not in the middle of experiencing overwhelming distress, they can usually explain what upsets them. Even young children often have ideas about where the problems are coming from. Listen to their concerns and try to understand their frustrations.

The first step to coming up with a solution is understanding what is causing the problem.

Some children may take more time to start talking than others will. Don't push or get frustrated with your child. If they really won't talk, you can always say, "It's OK. You can think about it, and we'll talk about it again later."

Another strategy some parents and High Em kiddos use is to give their strong emotions a name. For example, your child might call them Bert. This gives you and your child an easy way to talk about a challenging topic. "So what are we going to do when Bert shows up?" It puts you both on the same page against a common enemy. It removes blame from the child and focuses on that pesky disposition that gets the best of them. They hate it when Bert shows up too! Naming the wave of emotion sometimes helps High Em children when they feel their distress impulse activating. You can teach them to say, "I feel Bert coming on." It's another way to recognise and manage their emotions. It can help defuse the situation.

Books that talk about children dealing with strong emotions are another way you can help jump-start the conversation with your child. By reading about other children (or characters) who get really upset, your child learns that it's normal to feel angry, that the key is learning how to manage it. Focusing the discussion on an "other" can be less threatening, and may help your child ease into the topic. Further, books create an opportunity to explore different ways that children deal with their anger. Some examples of children's books that discuss anger include: *When I Feel Angry* by Cornelia Maude Spelman or *When Sophie Gets Angry–Really, Really Angry* by Molly Bang.

To open the problem-solving conversation with your child you can say, "I've noticed _____; what do you think is going on?" Name the problem as you see it. Phrase it as a challenge or a difficulty. For example, "I've noticed you have difficulty getting dressed in the morning; what do you think is going on?" "I've noticed that you find it challenging to stop doing what you're doing when I call you for dinner;

what do you think is going on?" Be patient and encouraging with your child. This is a chance for you both to express your concerns.

After you have each had a chance to talk about your concerns, say, "Let's think about how we can solve the problem. Do you have any ideas?" or "Let's think about how we can make things better. What are your ideas?"

Here's the hard part: you actually have to seriously listen to and consider each of your child's ideas. Some of them may be unrealistic, but don't immediately shut them down. Explain to your child that you have to come up with a solution that works for both of you. So if your child proposes eating chocolate for breakfast as a solution to morning meltdowns, you can say, "I like that you are coming up with ideas! But that one doesn't work for me because it's my role as a parent to make sure you eat a healthy breakfast. We need to find a solution that works for both of us. Let's think of some more ideas."

The flip side is that your child can also say that your idea doesn't work for them. Gulp. That's a hard one for parents, but that's collaborative problem-solving. I really wish my colleagues, my husband, and my friends would immediately recognise that my ideas are clearly the best ones, but alas, it turns out they often have their own ideas. Getting anything accomplished requires that we agree collaboratively on a way forward. If I try to impose my way, it's unlikely to result in any action. Trust me, I've tried. The dishwasher still doesn't get loaded to my specifications.

The same is true of your child. If you use problem-solving as a guise to actually implement your preconceived plan, your child will see right through it and lose faith in the process. It will be recognised as a sneaky way to unilaterally impose parental will and put you right back into a standoff with your High Em kiddo.

Keep in mind that the heart of the problem is that your child is not naturally disposed to manage strong emotions and handle challenging situations. Working through these problems with your child is likely to evoke strong emotions and be a challenging situation for *you* as the parent. As parents, raising our children is the one place we're used to being able to do things our way.

Ironically, that's exactly why problem-solving collaboratively with your child is effective. It teaches them how to manage strong emotions and work through challenging situations to come to a resolution. It teaches them to identify problems proactively, come up with ideas for how to tackle them, try them out, see how it goes, and adjust accordingly. It's actually a great rule book for life. Working collaboratively with your child, discussing each other's concerns, and then working together to find solutions also teaches your child the important skills of empathy and taking perspective.

Parents have asked whether young children can actually do collaborative problem-solving. The happy answer is yes! Children are like little scientists from a very young age—exploring and trying to understand their worlds (what happens when I push this juice off the table?). Once they are three or four, they have the ability to start to work with you on what's going on in their little heads when they get so upset. Of course, this ability will improve as they get older and their brains develop—up to a point. Teenagers seem to regress; sometimes it's easier to collaboratively problem-solve with my toddler (kidding, mostly)!

Put a plan in place. So you've talked with your child about the problem; you've each had a chance to express your concerns; and you have collaboratively come up with a solution that is mutually agreeable. It may not have been your first choice, but it's something. For example, perhaps the problem was that your child tended to throw tantrums on long car journeys. It was making trips to your parents' house miserable. Through your conversation, you learned that your child felt trapped and increasingly frustrated the longer he had to spend in the car. Your initial plan of offering a treat if the car trip went without a glitch hadn't worked; your High Em child simply didn't have the skill set yet to make it, even though he really wanted that treat. His suggestion that you no longer go on long car trips wasn't an option; you wanted to be able to take family trips to visit your parents. So, you problem-solved and came up with a plan to stop partway to take a break at the rest area playground. Not your first choice, because it makes a long trip longer, but if it works, it would be preferable to the kicking and screaming episodes that have become routine on family trips.

You have a plan. Now what?

Here's where the rubber meets the road. You try it out and see how it goes. Do not expect miracles. It will not be an overnight success. Because your child is genetically predisposed towards high Emotionality, it will require lots of practice, trial and error, and probably lots of failure as they work on developing their ability to manage strong emotions. Hang in there. Celebrate and reward little successes. This is a place where rewards *are* appropriate and effective for High Em children.

Keep an open line of communication with your child. When things don't go as planned, talk to them about what happened—but not in the moment. Do it when everyone is calm. "The plan for stopping on the way to Grandma's house didn't seem to help with your making the trip without getting upset. Why do you think that is?" "The plan didn't seem to help with getting out of the bath last night. What do you think happened?" Be encouraging of your child. Show them you believe in their ability to do better in the future. Remind them that it takes practice. They need your encouragement.

Think of it as developing a skill that your child doesn't naturally have. If they wanted to learn to play the piano, they couldn't just sit at the bench, start pressing keys, and immediately sound like Beethoven. It takes practice, and a lot of it. And you're going to have to deal with a lot of "Chopsticks" and bad music along the way.

If you find that you are seeing no improvement over the course of several weeks, then revisit the plan and come up with a new one together. Remind yourself that parenting is a marathon, not a sprint. My son is now thirteen. When I was in the thick of it, I admittedly had many days when I thought it would never end, but now we laugh together about the multitude of crazy emotional outbursts from his early childhood days.

Taking Care of Yourself

The reality is that children who are high on Emotionality—whose natural tendency is to respond with distress, frustration, or fear—pose a lot of challenges for parents. If you have a Low Em child, you lucked out on this front. You are likely to endure far fewer and far less extreme tantrums over the early years of your child's life. That's not to say there won't be challenges (there will), but your every request is less likely to be met with a stubborn "No!" or a thrown shoe. We've talked a lot about how all dispositions come with pluses and minuses; there are no "good" temperaments or "bad" temperaments. That's true, but the reality is that where children fall on Emotionality is strongly related to how "easy" parenting feels.

My hope is that reading this chapter will help parents of Low Em children better understand, and support, their parent friends who are struggling with High Em children. Your friends with children who are throwing astronomical fits aren't doing anything wrong. They aren't failing to implement proper rewards and consequences. It's not that their children need to learn appropriate behaviour. Their children just inherited a temperament towards really strong feelings, feelings that they are still learning to manage.

It's normal for parents of High Em children to feel especially frustrated, overwhelmed, and even resentful of their child at times. I went through five au pairs in two years. My best friend's nanny quit—on her birthday, no less—because she was embarrassed by the tantrums her daughter threw on the playground and the looks she got from the other children's parents. Raising High Em kids can be hard. Learning to let go of guilt related to having negative feelings towards your child is critical for your well-being, and for your ability to parent. Feelings of resentment don't mean you're a bad parent; they mean you're a human being, who doesn't like being yelled at or having your requests met with no response at best, or nasty reactions at worst. Having a High Em child can bring a lot of unanticipated stress into your home, and potentially your marriage.

That's why it's so important to take care of yourself. Parenting a High Em child takes extra patience, and it's especially hard if you're not in a good place mentally. There are great resources available for promoting well-being. One of my favourite is the Greater Good Science Center at the University of California, Berkeley (greatergood.berkeley.edu), which has a variety of science-based articles and tools. Mindfulness, meditation, yoga, taking long walks, exercising, finding joy in the small things. I know that it can be hard to take this advice seriously: Really? Like a bubble bath is going to make my child not destroy his room in a fit of rage? What exactly am I supposed to do with my screaming toddler while I am out taking long walks to smell the roses?

Children, especially challenging ones, can take up so much of our time and energy that it can feel like there's nothing left for ourselves. *But that's exactly why it's so important.* It is impossible to be a good parent if you don't take time for yourself. Taking care of others *requires* you to take care of yourself. Figure out what you need to recentre in order to have the patience you will need to work with your High Em child. Just like the process you've been doing to problem-solve with your child, pick one or two things to try, and work on implementing them. For example, maybe you used to love yoga, but have been too focused on battles with your child to find time anymore. Set aside one morning when you will get up thirty minutes early to have that time to yourself. Or perhaps you loved reading, but fall in bed exhausted now and can't remember when you last checked the *Sunday Times* Best Seller list. Order that book you've been wanting to read, and take ten minutes before bed for your own brief literary escape. Don't despair when you don't achieve your goal: when morning yoga gets interrupted by an early infant wake-up, or your bubble bath gets cut short by sibling squabbles, just take a deep breath and try again the next day.

Self-talk is a great way to help parents of High Em kids maintain their composure in the moment. Figure out your mantra and repeat it in your head while taking deep breaths when your child is having a meltdown. Here are some possibilities to get you started: "Life is just harder for some children." "They don't want to feel this way either." Or my personal favourite for truly astronomical meltdowns: "Love the child, blame the genes [breathe in, breathe out]. Love the child, blame the genes . . ." Whatever your mantra, it's a great coping mechanism.

Finally, although High Em kids don't always make it easy, don't forget to delight in their fiery spirit! You can lament the fact that they throw fits, or you can reframe their high Emotionality to focus on how it will serve them well in the future. Often the children we find most challenging to raise are the ones who grow up to be particularly interesting as adults. As eminent Pulitzer Prize–winning Harvard University professor Laurel Thatcher Ulrich wrote, "Well-behaved women seldom make history". It's true more broadly of all children. Some of the most challenging ones are the ones who change the world. Keep reminding yourself of that as they are stomping their feet or arguing back endlessly. Those strong emotions can be channelled towards a relentless pursuit of important passions as they get older.

Taking the Temperature on Your Own Emotionality

There's one last piece that influences how hard parenting is: where *you* fall on Emotionality. How naturally prone you are to distress, frustration, and worry will influence how much your child's behaviour upsets you. That's true whether you have a Low or High Em child. Parenting takes a lot of patience, and those of us who are higher on Emotionality are not naturally disposed to it! Our disposition towards distress can lead us to react strongly to our child's misbehaviour. That's not good for anyone. I know, I've been there.

The reality is that many of us can benefit from the same types of strategies we are trying to teach our children: taking deep breaths, concentrating on staying calm, figuring out a plan for how to deal with the strong emotions our children evoke, being kind to ourselves when we don't live up to our plan, and trying to do better next time. If you are high on Emotionality, don't be afraid to talk to your High Em child about it. Don't be afraid to use yourself as a model of someone who is also working on managing strong feelings. It will help your child understand that there is nothing "wrong" with them, and it will provide an opportunity to model the process of growth.

Siblings: It's Not Fair!

If you have more than one child, chances are they will differ on Emotionality. Having a child who is high on Emotionality can be difficult for their Low Em siblings. The outbursts may be frightening to them. Your High Em child may demand more of your time and energy. Your Low Em child may feel lost in the process. The fact that you may have to implement different parenting strategies for your children is likely to be perceived as unfair.

The key to navigating differences between siblings is to have open lines of communication in the family. As with differences in Extraversion, differences between siblings on Emotionality are a great opportunity to teach your children about empathy—about understanding that everyone is different, and valuing those differences. The parenting strategies that are key to working with High Em children teach your Low Em child valuable lessons too. You will be modelling the process of respecting others' opinions, openly discussing concerns, problem-solving solutions, and working together.

The reality is that siblings will always be treated differently. Your children may respond to differences in parenting as "not fair!" After all, they can only see the world through their own genetic lens, and their undeveloped brains can't fully comprehend that other brains work differently. But fair does not mean equal. If one child was disposed towards football and the other towards music, you would support each in excelling in their own way. If one child needs extra help with maths, you would give it to them—and not require the sibling who isn't struggling to sit in on maths tutoring sessions. Your children who differ on Emotionality will need different things from you, and that's OK. The best parenting is tailored to each child—no one size fits all.

Takeaways

- The most effective way to shape future behaviour in children is to work on promoting good behaviour rather than focus on punishing bad behaviour; but the strategies you implement need to be tailored to your child's Emotionality.

- For Low Em children, properly implemented rewards and consequences are highly effective in shaping their behaviour.

- Rewards should be enthusiastic, specific, immediate, and consistent. Focus on a small number of behaviours at a time and reward small steps in the right direction. Consequences should be used more sparingly, and will almost never "fit the crime". Cultivate the ability to "not sweat the small stuff".

- High Emotionality children frequently evoke harsh, negative responses from their parents, but these are the kids who need and benefit most from parental *warmth* and *gentle* discipline; typical parental consequences implemented at the time of outbursts often make the behaviour worse, not better.

- Focus on the *triggers* to extreme behaviour (temper tantrums, throwing objects, hitting) rather than on the *behaviour* itself.

- Reduce emotional outbursts by working with your child to identify the *why* behind their emotional reactions so that you can problem-solve with your child to come up with a plan to help them manage their strong emotions.

- Raising a High Em child can be challenging. Remember that parenting is a marathon, not a sprint, so you have to stay in shape! Take care of yourself so you have the mental energy to work with your High Em child.

CHAPTER 6

Effortful Control: The "Ef" Factor

In the 1960s, a team of researchers at Stanford University presented preschoolers with a choice: one treat now (for example, a biscuit, marshmallow, or other delicacy of their choosing) or two treats later. To get double the treats, they had to sit in a room, staring at the tempting treat for up to twenty minutes, waiting for the person conducting the experiment to come back, at which time they would get two treats. Children differed tremendously in whether they could wait to get the bigger reward, or whether they impulsively wanted their treat *right now*. The experiment famously came to be known as the Marshmallow Test.

The most fascinating part of the study is that the researchers continued to follow the children as they grew up. Whether the child could wait for the greater reward as a preschooler was predictive of all kinds of life outcomes. Children who could wait longer had higher SAT scores and better social and academic skills in adolescence. They gave in less to temptation, and were better able to concentrate, think ahead, and plan. In young adulthood, they used fewer drugs, achieved higher educational levels, and had lower body mass indexes (BMIs). They were better at handling stress and frustration, and did better at pursuing their goals.

The Marshmallow Test has been repeated around the world with similar results. Studies that have followed entire cohorts of children from early childhood to adulthood similarly find that self-control measured in young children is predictive of a host of life outcomes. For example, a famous longitudinal study conducted in New Zealand has followed a cohort of a thousand children born in the early 1970s for nearly five decades, starting at birth. The researchers found that childhood self-control was related to physical health, substance use problems, personal finances, and criminal offending, above and beyond children's intelligence and their social class. Self-control even predicted outcomes within families—with siblings who had lower self-control having poorer outcomes than their more controlled siblings.

How can something as simple as a child's ability to wait for a second marshmallow be so telling about future outcomes? And what does that mean for us parents who have children who most certainly would have marshmallow-stuffed cheeks?

The Marshmallow Test is predictive because it taps into a child's level of Effortful Control. Effortful Control refers to an individual's ability to regulate their behaviour, emotions, and attention. High Ef children can patiently wait to double their reward; low Ef children are enjoying the marshmallow before the researcher leaves the room!

Effortful Control goes by many names: self-control, behavioural control, impulse control. Children who are low on Effortful Control are called *impulsive* or *distractible*. Children who are high on Effortful Control are called *conscientious* or *dependable*. I prefer the term Effortful Control because (1) I like alliteration, and it's easier for me to remember the Big Three Es of children's dispositional styles (*Ex*traversion, *Emo*tionality, and *Ef*fortful Control), and (2) it emphasises that it takes *Effort*.

Self-control is hard! If it wasn't, then we would all keep our New Year's resolutions and be our fantasy selves by now. Because self-control is genetically influenced, it's harder for some people than others. Where we fall on Effortful Control starts with the luck of the draw when it comes to the genes we inherited. As the Marshmallow Test illustrates, differences in Effortful Control show up early in development, and they are stable. But the good news is that Effortful Control is also malleable. We can develop skills that don't come naturally to us, it just takes . . . effort. For those of us parents with marshmallow gobblers, it means that there is hope, that there are things we can do to help them develop more self-control.

The Brain Science Behind Effortful Control

The ability to effortfully control one's behaviour and emotions is related to two key areas of the brain. The first—the limbic system—has been called the *hot* brain. It is located deep in the brain, and is the most basic, primitive part. It is emotional, reflexive, and unconscious. It is highly tuned for "go!" responses. It quickly produces strong reactions to emotional stimuli, especially to pain, pleasure, and fear. It is also fully functional at birth; that's why babies are quick to cry when hungry or in pain. They don't need to learn how to get your attention when they are hurt or hungry. They know instinctively. It's highly evolutionarily adaptive that the hot brain is in place from the start. It's also why toddlers have so little self-control—they only have highly developed hot brains. They are like little engines with no brakes.

The brakes come from a second, more complex brain area—the prefrontal cortex. That's the part of your brain behind your forehead. The prefrontal cortex develops more slowly, and is not fully complete until the mid-twenties (with some evidence that it matures slightly later in boys as compared to girls, which comes as no surprise to us ladies). This "cool" part of the brain is involved in more reflective, complex decision-making. Interestingly, insurance companies "discovered" that brain development doesn't level off until the mid-twenties before scientists did; their databases showed that car accidents dropped off dramatically after age twenty-five. That's why insurance rates are so high for teenagers, and you can't hire a car until you're twenty-one in the UK and some hire companies impose higher insurance rates for those under twenty-five years old. As the prefrontal cortex reaches its full mature status, it enables complex, higher- order thinking like planning and decision-making, which helps keep our impulsive tendencies in check—all of which result in better drivers with fewer accidents.

More broadly, our prefrontal cortex helps us delay gratification and pursue long-term goals. It is the most intricate and highly developed part of the brain. All children show an increase in Effortful Control as they get older and their prefrontal cortex develops. But *how much* Effortful Control children develop is a product of their unique brain wiring.

Our natural dispositions towards Effortful Control are related to how active our "hot" brains are, as compared to our "cool" brains. In the Marshmallow Test, the kids who ate the marshmallow right away had brains that looked very different from the kids who waited for double the reward. The kids who opted to indulge in the immediate marshmallow had hot brain regions that were more active, especially in the presence of tempting stimuli. The parts of their brain that were attuned to pleasure, desire, and instant reward dominated. Conversely, the kids who could wait patiently for the greater reward had more active prefrontal cortexes—the cool brain region that controls planning and complex decision-making. In other words, the quick-to-eat-the-marshmallow kids had stronger engines, and the ones who waited for two marshmallows had stronger brakes.

The "hot" brain sometimes gets a bad rap, but it's important for a lot of reasons. It's the part of the brain involved in fight or flight. It makes quick decisions for us. It has been shaped by tens of thousands of years of evolution, and was critical for our ancestors to survive. In ancient times, it was a lot more important to be able to jump into action when confronted by a wild animal than it was to plan your ideal cave dwelling. We don't have to deal with a lot of surprise lion attacks these days, but we still need to make quick decisions to stay out of harm's way—to run when confronted by an intruder, to jump back from a snake, to duck when something is flying at you. Our brains serve us well when they can make reflexive, instantaneous decisions, rather than puzzling out all the possibilities. Our hot brains can save our lives.

Things that are important for survival and reproduction also produce hot brain reactions. Food and sex both produce rewarding feelings. Our hot brains like those feelings and seek them out more. It's what keeps us fed, and makes sure the human race continues generation after generation. Brains that are tuned to reward, to paying attention to present needs, are critical.

But responding to our immediate desires can also get us into trouble—especially in a world where there are lots of temptations. Our hot brains are biased towards the here and now, and there are a lot of here and now temptations in the world today. There is a lot of potential for immediate gratification. It's more fun to eat the biscuit now—but it may cause weight gain in the future. It's more fun to go out with friends, but it may interfere with getting homework done. It's more fun to sleep in than to go to the gym, but that won't help you be healthier in the long run. Overactivity in the hot brain region is related to obesity and addiction—disorders where controlling impulses plays a role. Our hot brain serves a lot of important functions, but it can also lead to problems.

That's where our "cool" brain comes into play. It helps us plan for the future and make hard decisions that help us achieve our long-term goals. Delayed rewards don't give us instant gratification, so they require thought. The hot brain says, "Eat the marshmallow!" But the cool brain says, "Wait, if I *don't* eat the marshmallow it will be better for me in the long run." The cool brain helps kids resist the temptation to jump on the sofa because you told them not to, and they will get into trouble if they do (even though it's so much fun . . .). As they get older, it's their cool brain that will help them say no to hanging out with friends so that they can study for their test the next day, so that they can get better grades, so that they can get into their preferred university, so they can get a better job, so they can have more financial stability . . . It's a complex process to think all that through—it's easier to let the hot brain say, "Yes, let's do it—party, here I come!"

Effortful Control is related to diverse positive life outcomes because the ability to plan ahead for the future helps us on lots of fronts. It helps us make hard decisions that delay gratification, but that result in larger rewards down the line. It allows us to pursue all kinds of different goals, whether they are related to health, family, school, or work. It stops us from doing things that will get us into trouble. Alas, our children start life with very little of it; their brains are simply not sufficiently developed yet.

Understanding the Many Faces of Effortful Control

How Effortful Control plays out in your child is related to where they fall on the other temperamental dimensions: Extraversion and Emotionality. Low Ef children who are also high on Extraversion are more impulsive and rowdy. They are the proverbial bulls in the china shop. They are the kiddos who think it's a great idea to jump out of the tree to impress their friends. And a quick peek into the future: because High Ex/Low Ef kids love being around people, and self-control doesn't come naturally to them, they are also more likely to get themselves into trouble as teenagers. As peers become increasingly important in adolescence, their hot brains are much more likely to spur them on to chase the fun. In teenagers, this means a higher likelihood to prioritise partying over studying, and increased likelihood of drinking and unprotected sex. Right now, though, you're more likely to have to worry about broken arms and A&E visits.

By contrast, Low Ef children who are high on Emotionality are especially prone to temper tantrums. They get upset easily and they struggle to control those strong feelings. In fact, because Emotionality involves one's ability to control emotions, it's not uncommon for High Em children to be low on Effortful Control. The silver lining is that as High Em/Low Ef children learn more Effortful Control strategies, their ability to manage their emotions will get better, and they will be better able to work with you on the collaborative problem-solving strategies we discussed in the last chapter. The natural maturation of their prefrontal cortex will also improve their Effortful Control, which will improve their ability to manage their emotions. Time is on your side.

Also keep in mind that people who are low on Effortful Control aren't necessarily low in all situations. They may have better self-control in some situations than in others. There are several different aspects of Effortful Control. Sometimes we need to get ourselves motivated to do something (get up and go to the gym), sometimes we need to get ourselves to stop (eating that extra piece of cake). Sometimes we have to stick with things that are boring (doing work, paying bills). And sometimes we have to keep ourselves from doing something we'll regret, either when we are in a really good mood (e.g. a night of overindulgence after a promotion), or in a really bad mood (e.g. telling off the boss). Children also vary in how their Effortful Control plays out across different settings.

In general, we overestimate how consistently we expect people to behave. Think back to the last chapter when we talked about how High Em children usually have particular situations that trigger their emotionality. They aren't highly emotional all the time. Low Ef individuals also usually have particular situations that are more challenging for them than others. For example, some Low Ef children have no problem completing homework, but they may have no control when it comes to jumping on the bed or racing through the house. Other Low Ef children may be generally good about following your directions—until they see something that excites them, and then they dart into the road to greet a friend.

You can think about challenges with Effortful Control as boiling down to two basic areas:

It's hard to STOP doing things we want to do (but shouldn't).
It's hard to START doing things we don't want do (but should).

STOP challenges are things like when your child is running wild at a birthday party, knocking over the decorations. START challenges are things like putting away toys at the end of a playdate.

Both of these challenges relate back to the fact that the present (what one wants right now) is more salient than the future (what might be best in the long run), especially for Low Ef children. Christopher is having so much fun running around at the party with friends that he is not thinking about how he is going to feel when the toy table gets knocked over. The embarrassment of a crash of packages as everyone stares at him, or his parent's scolding when that happens, is the furthest thing from his mind as he playfully tears around the room. Isabela is having so much fun with her dolls that she doesn't want to stop playing to put everything away and come downstairs for dinner. She is so focused on giving her baby a pretend bath that she isn't thinking about how cross her parent is going to be when they have to get up from the dinner table to collect Isabela from her room, only to discover baby clothes still covering the floor.

The good news is that if you have a Low Ef child, regardless of the area where they are struggling, a common set of strategies will help them learn more self-control. That's because all of the situations where Effortful Control is called for are assisted by *thinking about the future* and trying to *make it more present*. Some people can do this naturally and easily (High Ef individuals), but the rest of us need some additional tricks in our toolbox to practise self-control.

Strategies for Developing Effortful Control

The key to developing Effortful Control is to make it less effortful.

Remember that Low Ef kids have hot brain biases. Their brains lean towards the here and now. That means that when they fail to come when you call, or to stop running around when you ask, they aren't necessarily trying to be defiant or to ignore you. Their hot brains are wired to focus on the present, and their cool brains aren't proficient at thinking through the consequences for their future selves.

Helping your child develop more Effortful Control is about harnessing that basic insight and using it to work for them, instead of against them (and you). We're going to take advantage of their supercharged hot brain to help it do the cool brain's work. To do this, you have to trick their hot brains into paying more attention to the future, and less attention to the present moment. As Walter Mischel, the psychologist who designed the Marshmallow Test, put it: you want to heat the future, and cool the present. You bring the future to the here and now, where your Low Ef child lives. And you devise ways to manage the temptations of the present. We're going to walk through self-control strategies that focus on each of those pieces: making it less effortful, heating the future, and cooling the present.

Before we get started, here's bit of encouraging news for parents with Low Ef kiddos: the children who are the most genetically prone to having challenges with Effortful Control are also the ones who are most likely to benefit from intervention. In other words, the kids who have the lowest self-control are the ones who show the most improvement with self-control strategies. So let's jump in.

Make It Less Effortful

How do you make something easier that is, by definition, effortful?

You make it automatic.

When-Then plans are the key to making that happen. Part of what makes Effortful Control so hard (for ourselves and our children) is that in the moment, when we really want to do something (or not do something), our hot brains are dominating. For our Low Ef children, their undeveloped cool brains don't stand a chance at being able to reason them into what is best. When-Then plans eliminate the need for the cool brain to guide them to the better course of action. When-Then plans eliminate the need for thought altogether.

When-Then plans are simple: *when* X happens, *then* you will do Y. You let the hot brain, which registers the triggering situation, do the work. *When* my alarm goes off, *then* I will get out of bed. *When* my mum tells me to pull on my shoes, *then* I will pull on my shoes. You connect the situation that usually results in a breakdown of Effortful Control with a preplanned response. Every time the *When* happens, you respond with your *Then*. You don't think about it. You don't allow yourself to make any decisions in the moment. *When* X happens, *Then* do Y. Over time it becomes a habit and doesn't require Effortful Control anymore.

The key to success is to target a few of your child's behaviours that you really want to focus your effort on. The *When* can be almost anything. It can be an internal trigger (When I start feeling cross; When I get really excited) or an external trigger (When mum or dad asks me to come, When I see a dog on the street that I really want to pet). The *Then* is also anything you want to come up with. It will be situation dependent. The key is to have it be an action that is acceptable to you and your child and that solves the self-control challenge.

You can make When-Then plans for any situation where your child struggles with self-control, with the caveat that you can only focus on a couple at a time. You can't tackle all your child's self-control struggles at once (sorry). Remember that you are trying to remove the element of thinking things through, and if they have more than one or two When-Then plans that they have to try to remember, it's too much for their brains to develop that all-important automatic response.

The more your child rehearses and practices, the better they will get. *When* the green light goes on, *then* I can get out of bed. *When* I come inside, *then* I have to take off my shoes.

Start by making a list of the areas where your child struggles with Effortful Control. Remember that there are several ways that Low Ef can show up, since Effortful Control is about one's ability to control behaviour, emotions, and attention. Low Ef can manifest in different ways in different children. The table below lists some common areas where children struggle with self-control. Many of these situations are times when children feel strong emotions. Children can struggle with self-control when they are frustrated, angry, upset, bored, or alternatively, when they are feeling hyper or silly. Strong emotions tend to activate our hot brains, so it's not surprising that our ability to think rationally (i.e. use our cool brains) is compromised. It's true of all of us. I'm certainly guilty of shouting at my children when I'm actually frustrated that the repair man is an hour late.

COMMON SITUATIONS WHERE CHILDREN STRUGGLE WITH EFFORTFUL CONTROL
Trouble completing boring tasks (putting away toys, doing chores, brushing teeth, getting dressed, etc.)
Trouble managing strong emotions (anger, frustration)
Trouble stopping an activity to do something less "fun"
Risk-taking behaviour (e.g. jumping from high places, running into the sea)
Resisting temptations (e.g. a treat, something they are not supposed to touch)
Hyperactivity (running around the house, excessive energy when excited)

Remember that you can only work on a few things at a time. So pick the top one or two that are driving you most crazy (or, more generously, that are most concerning). You may have no problem generating the areas where your child struggles with self-control, or it may feel overwhelming to name them. Some parents tell me, "But there are so many, I don't know where to start!" Keeping a journal is always a good place to try to get a handle on your child's behaviour. Keep track of the areas where you see your child struggling with self-control, and then choose the ones that are most frequent, most troubling, or potentially dangerous to start with. If you're someone who usually has your phone in your pocket, you could make a quick note on your phone to help you track different events.

Once you have identified the areas where your child is having difficulty, work with your child to identify and name the triggers. You are essentially working with them on the *When*. Remember that the *When* can be an internal trigger (emotion) or an external trigger (something happens). Here are some examples:

- *When* my sibling makes me really cross
- *When* something happens that is unfair
- *When* I am feeling full of energy
- *When* my alarm goes off
- *When* my mum calls

Next come up with the *Then*. If your child's *When* is related to a strong emotion (anger, frustration), you want to choose a *Then* activity that will help them calm down (more on that later under "Have 'in-the-moment' cooling strategies"). It could be taking deep breaths, or going to their room for a quiet, calming activity (such as drawing or looking at a book). If their *When* is related to feeling full of energy or hyper, come up with a *Then* that will be an acceptable way to get that energy out without undesirable consequences:

- *Then* I will do jumping jacks
- *Then* I will take slow, deep breaths
- *Then* I will go to my room and colour

Your When-Then plan can also involve a "start" behaviour: *When* I call your name, *Then* you will put down what you are doing and come. *When* your sibling steals a toy, *Then* you will come tell me instead of hitting them. *When* I say it's time to clean your teeth, *Then* you will immediately go to the bathroom and brush. Your When-Then plan will be specific to the area you want to work on with your child.

Convey to your child that having a When-Then plan means *every time* the *When* happens, they must immediately do the *Then*. No questions asked. No exceptions.

The final piece is to reward them when they follow their When-Then plan. (You see why we discuss Effortful Control last—it brings everything together from the previous chapters!) Remember to reward them effusively and immediately: "Well done running up to brush your teeth right away when I asked!"

To give When-Then plans a jump start, you need to practise with your child. Have them pretend to be in the *When* situation, and practise immediately doing the *Then* response. Then reward and repeat. Remember that you're trying to make the behaviour automatic, and you do that by practising it time and time again. It helps the brain wire a new connection between *When* and *Then*.

For example, if your child's When-Then is *When* my mum calls, *Then* I will immediately stop what I am doing and go to her, have your child go to their room and pretend to be playing with their toys, call their name, and have them practise stopping everything right away and coming to you. If they are willing, try to get them to overexaggerate the behaviour. For example, if your daughter is in the middle of playing house, she can immediately drop all her family pieces and run to you. If your son is playing sword fighting, he drops his weapon in midair and heads your way at lightning speed. Reward with cheerleader-level praise. "Look how fast you came! Wow!"

If your child's When-Then is *When* I get really cross, *Then* I am going to take five long, slow breaths, then have them practise that. Come up with an imaginary scenario that relates to something that caused them to lose their temper in the past. Tell them to imagine how they are feeling: "You feel yourself getting more and more cross, like you might explode." Then you remind them of their *Then* behaviour. As soon as they have practised, immediately reward. Make it fun. Remember, hot brains like pleasure, so connecting their When-Then sequence to good feelings will help to solidify the behaviour.

You will notice many parallels between the When-Then strategy and the problem-solving strategies that we discussed in the last chapter for High Em children. When-Then strategies can be applied to any kind of self-control challenges, not just controlling emotions. They work equally well for children who struggle to control their behaviour, or to control their attention.

Making the Future More Hot

Another trick to help with Effortful Control is to make negative future consequences more immediate. Your child doesn't immediately stop playing with their toys and put on their pajamas when you ask, because they are focused on the present fun. They aren't thinking ahead ten minutes into the future when you are going to storm into their room and be really angry to discover no progress towards bedtime. Remember, hot brains focus on the present. Accordingly, you want to get your child to focus *now* on the future consequence. To help them with that, you need them to imagine how it is going to feel in the future *as if it is the present*.

Adults can do this pretty well by imagining it. When your spouse asks you to come help them with something, even though you may not want to, there is that little voice in your head that tells you it would be really rude to ignore them and you don't want to get into a fight. That's your prefrontal cortex working for you—your cool brain helps you think through the chain of logical future consequences. If you're trying to motivate yourself to get the laundry done, even though you might really want to watch another episode of *Modern Family*, you think about how annoying it will be when no one has clean underwear tomorrow.

But kids—especially Low Ef kids—can't do that complex future thinking. So you have to help make the future consequences more salient to the here and now. You have to create more emotion connected to the future consequence. You can do that by role-playing with them. Role-playing helps bring out the strong negative emotions associated with making a poor choice, to remind your child they don't want to go there. It gives them an "emotional preview", which activates their hot brains.

Here's how this might work: let's return to Isabela, who has trouble stopping playing with her toys when her parent calls. Mum or dad sits down to have a conversation with Isabela about this challenging behaviour and what they are going to do about it. They devise a When-Then plan. But then they say, "Let's imagine what happens when you don't stop playing with your toys." Isabela will probably offer, "Mum/dad gets *really cross*." "That's right," Mum says. "So let's pretend that happens." Mum has Isabela pretend she's playing with her toys; she calls her name and Isabela keeps right on playing (as they have schemed). So mum pretends to storm into her room and uses her actual serious cross voice to tell Isabela how upset she is, and she implements whatever consequence would normally result: "Young lady, I have told you it is unacceptable to ignore me when I call! Now go to the steps for time-out."

Another example could be to have your older child imagine that they were supposed to be in their room doing homework, but they started playing on their phone instead. You can pretend to walk into the room and find them on their phone and use your stern voice to say, "You told me you were doing your homework, but you played on your phone instead. Now you can't go over to your friend's house later because you have work to finish". The key is that you want to remind your child that it feels really rubbish when they don't listen. They don't like feeling that way. They don't like the consequence. By role-playing, you are making the consequence more real and immediate.

Critically, it's important to follow up this role-playing with practising your When-Then plan for this scenario. Then you can heap lots of praise on your child when she performs the desired response. "Wonderful! You came right away when I called!" "Great, you finished your homework before you started playing!"

In case you're thinking, "Isn't it mean to pretend to be cross at your child?!" remember that they know you are pretending. Even so, the role-play will still elicit an emotional response, which will help them learn to effortfully control their behaviour in the future. It's better to have a pretend consequence when they are learning with you than a real one when everyone is upset. And the When-Then practice, followed by praise that you do afterward, will end things on a positive note. In addition, the contrast (it feels bad when I don't pay attention to what I'm supposed to do; it feels good when I do) will reinforce the point that their choices can result in very different outcomes. It helps your child learn to effortfully control the outcome. It's a critical life skill that you are teaching them. Your child is learning that they are in charge of their life outcomes through the choices they make. You can't make those choices for them (as much as we want to), but this is how you start nudging them towards making good decisions.

Making the Now More Cold

The other way to build Effortful Control is to use strategies that cool down the need for it in the present moment. Here are some techniques:

Remove the temptation. This is a method that many of us use, both on ourselves and our children. The idea is to arrange our environments so that we have fewer triggers around us. For example, I don't buy crisps, because I find it nearly impossible not to eat the entire bag. We don't leave the biscuit tin sitting out in our family, because we know our children will see it and start whining for a biscuit. If you know your child will beg to stop at the playground and there's no time, choose a different route home from school that doesn't pass by. It's hard to avoid temptation when it's so front and centre. It's especially hard for people who are Low Ef. Removing temptations is perhaps one of the easiest ways to reduce self-control struggles, but it can only be useful in certain situations. Sometimes there's a big bowl of crisps inches from you at a party! Your child will face similar environments that are out of their control. And so, ultimately, you need to build your child's self-control muscle.

Create distraction. When removing temptation isn't an option, distraction is another great technique. We do this a lot with our kids. They start whining for something, and we say, "Oh, look, pavement chalk—let's go draw a picture!" Redirecting attention away from the tempting object is always a good option, especially for very young children, for whom When-Then strategies might still be challenging. Bottom line: if you can avoid the *When* (the triggering situation), that's often easiest. The preschoolers in the marshmallow experiments used a number of hilarious distracting techniques which you can find on YouTube, including looking away, drumming their fingers, making funny faces, or tapping their feet—anything to keep their mind off that marshmallow!

Try the "Fly on the Wall" technique. Learning how to step back from one's feelings and observe them from a distance is a core part of many therapies and practices that effectively decrease distress and increase well-being. It is a central part of cognitive behavioural therapy, one of the most effective therapies for many psychological challenges. It's also central to mindfulness, for which there is mounting evidence of its many benefits. Learning to remove yourself from the intensity of your feelings and observe them more objectively helps you get over the immediacy of strong, challenging emotions.

Our children also experience strong, challenging emotions (oh, don't they ever!). Teaching them to step outside themselves and reflect on the situation is one way to help them learn to manage their feelings and increase their Effortful Control. With kids, you can ask them to imagine that they are a fly on the wall watching the situation unfold. Generally this does not help in the moment, but it is good for "debriefing" the situation. Here's what this might look like:

> PARENT: "Let's try to figure out what happened when we got into that argument over getting ready for bed last night. Imagine you're a fly on the wall in your room; tell me what the fly saw."

Help guide your child through the conversation. There's no right way to do it, but the key is that you want your child to talk objectively through what each person was doing and feeling—i.e. try to cover each person's behaviours and emotions.

PARENT: "What is the fly watching you do?"

CHILD: "I'm playing with my toys."

PARENT: "And what am I doing?"

CHILD: "You're calling up to my room, telling me to put on pajamas."

PARENT: "And what does the fly see you doing after that?"

CHILD (*smiling sheepishly*): "I'm still playing with my toys."

PARENT: "Then what happened?"

CHILD: "You come into the room."

PARENT: "And what does the fly see Mum doing?"

CHILD: "shouting!"

PARENT: "How does Mum seem to be feeling?"

CHILD: "Cross."

PARENT: "Why do you think Mum is so cross?"

CHILD: "Because I didn't do what she asked."

PARENT: "What does the fly see next?"

CHILD: "I start shouting back."

You can try to infuse humour: "Wow, that fly sure landed in the wrong place; he had to listen to a lot of shouting!"

The point of the Fly on the Wall exercise is that it helps your child learn to take multiple perspectives. It moves them off their own viewpoint (which, let's be honest, many of us can get stuck in) and helps them see both sides. Research has shown that stepping back and trying to observe a situation in the third person helps children (and adults) get over angry or hurt feelings. It helps them to move on. It has been shown to work for both boys and girls, and children of all backgrounds. We all benefit from having some perspective.

Have "in-the-moment" cooling strategies. It's always a good idea to have some calming strategies ready for moments when Effortful Control is called for, but your child just isn't feeling it (their version of "Serenity now!" for the *Seinfeld* fans out there). We need these strategies as parents, and children need them too. Give them a go-to technique that they can easily summon when they feel a loss of Effortful Control coming on. It can be part of their When-Then plan. Cooling strategies can include: taking deep breaths, counting to ten, or squeezing their hands tight like they are squeezing lemons. They can also include things like asking to take a break, or having a go-to soothing, quiet activity (reading, colouring, listening to music) that will help them regain control. Figure out what resonates with your child. My child, for example, hated the idea of squeezing his hands like lemons; he felt it looked ridiculous and it actually made him more worked up, not less. Instead, he found that going to his room and sitting on a bean bag by himself was a much better way for him to calm down and regulate himself.

Other Things Parents Can Do to Help Children Build Effortful Control

So far we've talked about specific strategies you can implement to work on particular areas where your child is struggling with self-control. But there are also some general areas that you can influence as a parent that are known to impact children's ability to effortfully control their behaviour.

Eat, sleep, and be merry. Everyone has better self-control when they are not tired or hungry—this is true for both kids *and* adults. On some level, we all know this, but sometimes it's the simplest things that get overlooked. Healthy sleeping and meal habits keep us all at our best. Having your child stick to the same bedtime and waketime, creating a standard evening routine, and avoiding stimulating activities or screen time right before bed are all ways to help promote well-rested children, who wake up ready to be on their best behaviour (smile). Foregoing that last errand that you really want to squeeze in when everyone is "over" shopping, making sure meals don't get skipped, and keeping healthy snacks in the car for emergencies (I have a whole stash in my glove box—mostly for me) are all ways to promote smoother days.

Monitor stress levels. Stress can have a tremendous impact on brain development. Stress puts us into fight-or-flight mode. It does this by activating the "hot" system of the brain. Children who grow up in a state of constant stress have "hot" brain systems that are overactive and on high alert. This makes it harder for children to learn to control their impulses and to develop Effortful Control. When the world is unpredictable and dangerous, evolution has primed our hot brains to take over.

Accordingly, as a parent, one of the most important things you can do is to help your child feel safe, secure, and loved. To the extent that it is under your control, you can help their world be more stable and predictable. Intense arguing or domestic violence in the home, adults who are untrustworthy, neighbourhoods that are dangerous—all these things can make it difficult for children to nurture their ability to think and plan. Instead, they are forced to attend to the here and now. To the extent that parents are able to help reduce sources of chronic, high stress in their children's lives, children benefit.

Encourage autonomy. Reducing stress does not mean you should try to control every aspect of your child's environment. In fact, being too protective of your child also hurts their ability to develop Effortful Control. Parents need to support and encourage autonomy. Children build their Effortful Control skills by trying things out and learning from consequences. Just as with taking their algebra test, mastering self-control isn't something parents can do for them. Kids have to learn for themselves. In contrast to algebra, Effortful Control skills are likely to be far more important to their life outcomes! So give them opportunities to practise and build their Effortful Control. They won't always get it right. But they will get better at it.

For example, your child might ask if they can play a game before starting their homework. You are doubtful that they will be able to pull themselves away from the game to switch gears into work mode. Allowing them to try, however, will give them the opportunity to practise their Effortful Control skills. You might be pleasantly surprised. Minimally, by giving your child a chance, you avoid the pushback, arguing, and resentment that can come from setting the boundaries for them. And if they don't rise to the occasion, then your child will learn that this is an area they still need to work on; it creates an opportunity for a collaborative conversation with your child about building self-control.

Allow natural consequences. One of the ways that children learn self-control is by experiencing consequences. That can be hard for parents, as it feels like part of our role is to protect our children. But by "protecting" them from the consequences of their actions, we actually harm them in the long run, since their brains don't make the cause-and-effect connections between their behaviour and their outcomes. For example, if your child is fooling around in the morning and forgets their school bag, don't take it to school for them. One day without their books is not the end of the world, and experiencing that discomfort will make them more likely to stay focused on gathering their school supplies in the future. Children need to learn that choices have consequences, and that they can choose. By allowing consequences to play out, children learn that good choices lead to good consequences, and bad choices lead to bad consequences. Help them make the connection between their behaviour and the consequence (for better or worse), so they start to develop this basic insight and realise that they have the power to affect the outcome.

Know when to implement damage control. There are certain tasks that simply exceed some children's ability to exert Effortful Control, and for which allowing natural consequences isn't an option. If your child has very little self-control in a particular area that could lead to problems, sometimes the most prudent course of action is to expect that they will not have the necessary self-control for the task at hand, and figure out how to minimise collateral damage. This is why we build fences around pools, and why you keep a close eye on your toddler at the beach. Small children (or Low Ef children) don't have the self-control to reliably make good decisions (for example, they don't think through the fact that they can't swim before running into the water). Sometimes our role as parents is simply to protect them, and to not expect that they will rise to the challenge. This can also apply to smaller, non–life-threatening self-control tasks as well. My developmental psychology faculty colleague has a daughter who went through a phase when she was about a year old where she routinely threw her food. Knowing that impulse control was still outside of her daughter's developmental mastery, their family simply moved the kitchen table to the far side of the room so that all upholstered furniture was outside the line of fire while they slowly worked with her on keeping her food on her plate.

Provide examples of Effortful Control. Children learn by observing, and because all children have brains that are still developing Effortful Control (some faster than others, you lucky parents of High Ef children!), there are a lot of resources out there to help kids learn self-control. If you google "self-control books for kids", you will come up with hundreds of stories you can read with your child that are designed to help them develop an understanding of self-control. If you are a good storyteller, you can create tales about fictional children who vary in self-control. The 2013 and 2014 seasons of *Sesame Street* were developed in consultation with Walter Mischel, the Marshmallow Test psychologist, and focus on helping children learn self-control strategies as they watch Cookie Monster learn to control his cookie cravings. Vivid storytelling can slowly help children connect behavioural choices with outcome.

Play games that practise Effortful Control. Many popular games for children actually help them develop self-control. In Red Light, Green Light, the child can only move forwards from the starting line towards the finish line when the leader says "Green Light", but has to stop moving when they say "Red Light". Children who are still moving after the "Red

Light" command have to go back to the starting line. In the game "Simon Says," children must act out whatever command the player designated "Simon" says (e.g. "Simon says touch your nose." "Simon says jump on one foot.") but only when prefaced by the phrase "Simon says". If the Simon player simply says, "Touch your nose" and the child carries out the action, they are eliminated from the game. Each of these games allows children to practise impulse control—and the best part? Kids are having fun, and not even aware that they're practising self-control skills!

Model Effortful Control. Children also learn a lot about Effortful Control by observation, and they get a front-row seat in observing their parents. When our children push our buttons, how do we respond? When we experience strong feelings, those emotions can activate our hot brains and lead us to act reactively, rather than thoughtfully. Just like our kids, we all differ in how naturally Effortful Control comes to us. It's worth reflecting on the areas where self-control may be more challenging for you. Think about your triggers, particularly as they relate to your child. It's good to have a plan in place for how you will respond when your child challenges your Effortful Control. The good news is that all the techniques we have covered work for adults too. When-Then plans, cooling strategies, learning to step back from one's feelings—these are all methods we can use to help us be better, calmer parents.

I will confess that there are times when I let my hot brain take over when dealing with my son. We all have moments when our Effortful Control runs low. A close friend recently told me about how at the end of a long, quarantine day with her children, she was checking the homework her daughter was supposedly working on all day, only to discover it was blank. After a heated, convoluted exchange about how maybe possibly the computer had failed to save her work, my friend finally screamed out a less polite version of: *"Just tell me where the heck your homework is!"*

Sometimes we are not our best selves in spite of our best-laid plans. That's just life, and it's an important lesson for your child to learn too.

If you find yourself losing control and having an outburst you later regret, be honest with your child about it. Talk to them about what happened (once everyone is calm again), just as you would if *they* had a breakdown in Effortful Control. You can use it as an opportunity to remind them that we all make mistakes; that when we do, we apologise; and then we all move on and try to do better in the future. This is a way that you can model the process of developing Effortful Control that you want your child to learn.

Is It Possible to Have Too Much Self-Control?

In general, Effortful Control is a good thing; it is associated with many positive life outcomes, as we have discussed in this chapter. But at times children who are very high in Effortful Control can be "overcontrolled". Their disposition towards being in control may lead them to be too cautious, and unwilling to take any risks. Overcontrolled children can also be rigid and inflexible. They may have trouble when there are changes in plans. This high degree of self-control may lead to conflict with other children who are not as rule-oriented, causing challenges with peers.

If your High Ef child displays any of these tendencies, you can work with them on the areas where they are struggling. Gently challenge your cautious child to try something new. Start small, and praise them for stepping out of their comfort zone. If your child's inflexibility is causing problems, try using the problem-solving strategies we discussed in chapter 5 about Emotionality. If they are frustrated by other children who don't have the same level of self-control, use it as an opportunity to talk to them about individual differences, and how there are good aspects and drawbacks to all characteristics, including things like risk-taking. Have them think through the pros and cons with you, so they better appreciate different ways of being.

Should You Ever Eat the Marshmallow?

As you have been reading this chapter you may have been thinking, "But why is it such a bad thing to gobble down the marshmallow?" After all, *carpe diem*, seize the day!

It turns out that there are actually situations where it makes sense to take advantage of opportunities that are directly in front of you. When your environment is unpredictable, or it is uncertain whether people will keep their word about future rewards, it makes sense to take advantage of the proverbial bird (or marshmallow!) in the hand. In fact, in the Marshmallow Test, the researchers found that children were more likely to wait if they'd had experience with other people following through on what they said they would do. If there's no reason to believe that someone will deliver on their promise of two marshmallows at a later time, then it makes sense to eat the one marshmallow when you have the chance.

There are also times when jumping on opportunities as they arise can be advantageous. CEOs and other leaders tend to be higher on certain dimensions of impulsivity like risk-taking. Taking too much risk, however, can be disastrous. Quickly following what feels right in the moment can get us into a lot of trouble. It leads people to use drugs, gamble, have unprotected sex, eat the entire bag of crisps. There are many situations where doing what we want in the moment is not the best thing for us in the long run. So, yes, while some degree of risk-taking and jumping on opportunities can be a good thing, the key is to find the right balance and learn to take *calculated* risks. And that's where Effortful Control comes in. It doesn't eliminate the advantages associated with being a risk-taker, it just helps one control it.

Gender Differences

We haven't talked much about gender differences in the previous chapters. That's because for most temperamental dispositions there really aren't any. Effortful Control is the exception. As a group, girls score much higher on Effortful Control than boys (as any mum of boys could have told you!). This also validates the repeated observation that in school settings, girls are generally perceived as more focused and compliant, exhibiting greater self-control. They can sit attentively in their seats for longer and are better about completing their assignments. Disorders that are related to impulse control (e.g. ADHD and aggression in kids, substance use problems in adulthood) are also higher in boys than in girls. It's unclear whether these mean-level differences in behavioural control are due to biological or societal differences. Like most things, it's probably a combination of both. It's also important to remember that even though *on average* girls show higher levels of Effortful Control than boys, both sexes have a bell-curve–shaped distribution, meaning that some girls and boys are at the low or high ends, and a lot are in the middle.

Summing Up

All kids struggle with self-control. They hit their sibling right after they promise you they won't. They ignore your requests to tidy up, and keep right on playing with their toys. They kick the football in the house and break your new lamp. Lapses in self-control are the top of the list of things-our-kids-do-that-drive-us-crazy.

Part of the reason it is so frustrating is because it feels like our kids *should* be able to behave, and they are choosing not to. After all, they have just told you "hands are not for hitting" or "sharing is caring". This is called the *expectation gap*, or the idea that parents believe their children are capable of more Effortful Control, at a younger age, than the research on brain development indicates is possible. In other words, just because your child can dutifully (even genuinely) recite the rule for you does not mean that their brains have the ability to follow through on it. Their hot brains are fully functional, but their cool brains have a long way to go. That makes it incredibly hard to control impulses. On top of that, their individual brain is programmed differently, depending on its unique genetic code. Low Ef kids will have hot brain biases that stretch across their lives.

This chapter covered strategies that help kids learn more Effortful Control, but they are not magic. When-Then plans can target the high priority areas, but remember that you're working against thousands of years of evolutionary programming. Your child's brain is wired to respond to the here and now, especially if you have a Low Ef child. It takes time to make a behaviour automatic, and even when your child builds their Effortful Control, they will still slip up from time to time.

That's when it's up to us parents to practise our Effortful Control. Take a few deep breaths and remind yourself that their brains are under construction. That basic insight—that they are not wilfully being bad; their brains are just still under development—can be a go-to cooling strategy for you. It certainly helped me maintain my sanity when my toddler got out of his chair for the tenth time after I'd repeatedly told him to stay seated. It also underscores why lecturing, or even shouting at, children isn't an effective way of teaching Effortful Control. Alas, it won't make their brains grow any faster, and punishing them for failing to behave in ways that are beyond their capacity only makes them feel bad about themselves. In the marshmallow experiment, most children under the age of four couldn't wait for the second marshmallow—and some kids will always be predisposed to go for the immediate treat. Keep nudging them towards Effortful Control, even when they push yours to the limit!

Takeaways

- Effortful Control refers to an individual's ability to regulate their behaviour, emotions, and attention. It is genetically influenced, with differences showing up early in development, but it is also malleable.

- The ability to effortfully control behaviour is related to the development of two key brain areas, referred to as the *hot brain* (limbic system) and *cool brain* (prefrontal cortex). The hot brain focuses on the here and now; the cool brain is involved in decision-making and planning.

- The cool brain takes a long time to develop; that's why most children struggle with self-control in some form or another. Low Ef children have hot brain biases that persist even as they get older.

- Several strategies can help children develop more Effortful Control. These include When-Then plans, role-playing consequences, and cooling strategies.

- Remembering that your child is not trying to be defiant, that their brain is just biased to the here and now, can help you be more patient (and practise more Effortful Control!) with your child.

CHAPTER 7

* * * ▬▬▬ * * *

Beyond You and Your Child: Predispositions and Partners

A t this point you have a good understanding of your child, their natural tendencies, and how their brain works. And you have a better understanding of yourself, your natural tendencies, and how your brain works. You have learned how to use this knowledge to create Goodness of Fit–flexibly adapting your parenting to your child's needs to help them grow into their best selves, and reducing unnecessary stress and battles at your house.

But you are probably not the only important adult in your child's life. Other important adults in your child's life—co-parents, significant others, caregivers, grandparents, teachers, coaches—also play a role in creating Goodness of Fit. They probably have their own ideas about parenting and how best to shape and discipline children. In this chapter, we'll walk through how to have conversations to create Goodness of Fit with other important individuals in your child's life, and how to address differences in parenting styles and beliefs across caregivers. The first part of the chapter covers conversations with co-parents, a term which I use here broadly to refer to any other important adult playing a role in parenting your child. The second part of the chapter is specifically devoted to the school setting and developing partnerships with teachers.

The information in this second part of the chapter can also be applied to having conversations with coaches and other part-time caretakers who play important roles in your child's life, such as babysitters.

Navigating Co-Parenting

If you are married or partnered, your spouse/significant other is in all likelihood the other person playing a big role in disciplining your child and dealing with the day-to-day. And if you are like many couples, you may not share exactly the same parenting philosophy. If you are no longer married or in a relationship with your child's other biological parent, coming to agreement about parenting can be even more challenging. In some families, other important adults reside in the home, such as grandparents or extended family members, and those individuals also play a role in child-rearing. Throughout this section I use the word *partner* to encompass these many types of other adult individuals who may be participating in parenting your child.

So what do you do when other important adults in your child's life have very different ideas about parenting? Maybe they were raised with strict discipline and think the idea of adapting to children's needs is some New Age version of being soft. Maybe they have strong ideas about the "right" way to parent and don't believe in flexibly adapting parenting to the child. (I might suggest you give them a copy of this book to read as a starting point.) Maybe your High Em child is acting out and your partner is telling you that your child just needs more discipline. Maybe your partner thinks that your lack of rules is contributing to your child's outbursts or unacceptable behaviour. It's not uncommon for one parent to think the other is too permissive, while the co-parent views the other parent as too strict or uncompromising. How do you navigate these differences, which can be yet another source of stress in your home?

Let's start by stepping back and reviewing the research on parenting styles.

Understanding Your Parenting Style

Psychologists talk about parenting styles as falling along two key dimensions: warmth (which involves responsiveness) and control (which encompasses demandingness and strictness). Each is a continuum, with parents ranging from high to low on each dimension. Where parents fall on these two dimensions creates four different parenting "styles," which have been labelled Authoritative, Permissive, Uninvolved, and Authoritarian.

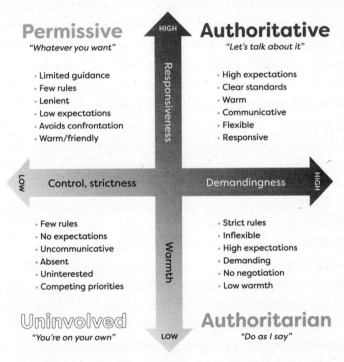

Permissive
"Whatever you want"

- Limited guidance
- Few rules
- Lenient
- Low expectations
- Avoids confrontation
- Warm/friendly

Authoritative
"Let's talk about it"

- High expectations
- Clear standards
- Warm
- Communicative
- Flexible
- Responsive

HIGH — Responsiveness

LOW — Control, strictness — Demandingness — HIGH

Warmth — LOW

- Few rules
- No expectations
- Uncommunicative
- Absent
- Uninterested
- Competing priorities

- Strict rules
- Inflexible
- High expectations
- Demanding
- No negotiation
- Low warmth

Uninvolved
"You're on your own"

Authoritarian
"Do as I say"

Source: Fernando García and Enrique Gracia. "Is Always Authoritative the Optimum Parenting Style? Evidence from Spanish Families." *Adolescence* 44, no. 173 (Spring 2009): 101–31.

Authoritative parents are high on warmth, and high on demandingness. They are parents who set high expectations and have clear standards for their children, and communicate those expectations in a warm manner. They set rules and explain the reasoning behind rules. They allow children to have input into goals and activities.

187

Permissive parents are also high on warmth, but they offer more limited guidance or direction for their children. They have fewer rules, and are more lenient when their children break the rules. Permissive parents are more likely to want to be their child's friend. They are not as strict, and tend to let their children figure things out for themselves. They are warm and nurturing, but do not set high expectations for their children to follow.

Authoritarian parents are high on demandingness like Authoritative parents, but they are not as high on warmth. They tend to set and enforce strict rules for their children, with little input from the child. Their rules are inflexible, and breaking the rules results in punishment. Negotiation with the child is viewed as unacceptable. Communication tends to be one-way: from parent to child, and the child is expected to follow rules without questioning. Authoritarian parents tend to be less warm and nurturing.

Uninvolved parents are low on warmth and demandingness. These parents tend to let their children do what they want with little direction and few boundaries. Communication is rare. There are few rules or expectations. These parents are absent or consumed with other priorities. At the extreme, Uninvolved parents are neglectful.

Let's look at how these parenting styles play out in a few typical parenting situations:

Five-year-old Ethan is shopping with his mother. Ethan feels like it is taking a really long time and he becomes frustrated. He throws his juice box down, which proceeds to splatter all over the floor. Here's how parents with different types of parenting styles might respond:

THE AUTHORITATIVE PARENT *(In a Firm But Gentle Voice)*: "Ethan, I know you are tired of shopping, but we need to go to the shops so that we have food in the house for dinner. What have we talked about with respect to throwing? It's not OK to throw things when you're angry. Now, what are you going to do about the spilled juice on the floor?"

THE PERMISSIVE PARENT (*gives Ethan a mischievous look*): "Ethan, you know you shouldn't do that. But I know shopping is boring. Let's finish up shopping and get home, and I'll make you dinner."

THE AUTHORITARIAN PARENT (*raises voice and speaks harshly*): "Ethan, that is absolutely unacceptable! You are going to your room as soon as we get home, and no pudding!"

THE UNINVOLVED PARENT: Doesn't notice that Ethan threw down the juice box.

Fast-forward ten years. Here's another scenario. Fifteen-year-old Ethan comes home past his midnight curfew:

THE AUTHORITATIVE PARENT: "Ethan, we've talked about your curfew and you know it is midnight. It's not acceptable for you to be thirty minutes late for no good reason. As we have discussed, because you came home late, you won't be allowed to go out with your friends tomorrow night. Let's think through some ways you can keep track of the hour better the next time."

THE PERMISSIVE PARENT: "Ethan, try not to be late next time."

THE AUTHORITARIAN PARENT (*raises voice*): "Ethan, it is unacceptable to be late! What were you thinking? It is not OK to disobey me. You're grounded until I say otherwise."

THE UNINVOLVED PARENT: Ethan doesn't have a curfew.

In reading through the above scenarios, you likely recognise parts of yourself in some of the possible parenting responses. What kind of parenting style do you tend to use? You probably identify most closely with one of the above styles, although you may see elements of yourself across each of the styles. You may also find yourself adopting different parenting styles in different situations, or with different children, or at different times in your children's lives. This is because children's behaviour often drives parental responses, as we discussed in chapter 1. For example, High Em children may start to evoke more Authoritarian parenting as parents initially try to clamp down on "bad" behaviour. That may be followed by more Permissive parenting as parents start to give up because seemingly nothing is working.

Authoritative parenting is the style that is thought to be most beneficial for child development. Authoritative parents set appropriate boundaries and limits for their children, while also nurturing an ability for children to learn from their mistakes and think for themselves. Authoritative parenting, characterised by both warmth and control, has been associated with a number of positive child outcomes across countless studies, including higher levels of academic performance and social competence, and lower levels of aggression, anxiety, and depression, and fewer behavioural problems.

Let's unpack the Authoritative parenting response to little Ethan's juice-throwing tantrum and see why it is particularly helpful for child development. "Ethan, I know you are tired of shopping [*shows empathy with the child and acknowledges their feelings*], but we need to go to the shops so that we have food in the house for dinner [*reiterates what they have to do and explains why the activity is necessary*]. What have we talked about with respect to throwing? It's not OK to throw things when you're angry [*reminds the child that they have talked about this issue before and what the family rule is*]. Now, what are you going to do about the spilled juice on the floor? [*Holds the child responsible for their action and making it right, without being pejorative. Treats the inappropriate behaviour as a mistake, not a reflection of the child being bad. Involves the child in coming up with a solution to their mistake.*]

Of course, how one handles one episode of juice throwing in the supermarket is not going to make or break a child. And we've all had moments when we are not our best parenting selves. My child has definitely pushed and whined and pestered until I finally snapped back, "Because I'm the parent and I said so!" (which displays *none* of the good

Authoritative parenting qualities). But in general, there is a lot of research suggesting that adopting a consistent Authoritative parenting style is associated with a range of positive child outcomes.

It's Not All About You

But here's the wrinkle. The way we view parenting is a reflection of our own unique genetically influenced temperamental styles. This is true of everyone taking part in the parenting process: dispositions influence the way *our children* view our parenting, the way *we view ourselves* as parents, the way *we view our partner's* parenting, and the way *our partners view* our parenting. Our unique genetic dispositions also influence the way we perceive our children's behaviour and how problematic, or not, we view certain behaviours.

Let's unpack these different pieces. First, you and your partner may not agree on whether your child's behaviour is problematic. In child development research it's not uncommon for researchers to have multiple people report on a child's behaviour—parents, teachers, and other care-givers. And a consistent finding is that the adults in a child's life don't always agree about that child's general behaviour. This could be partly because children behave differently around different people and in different settings. I was always taken aback when my son's friends' parents would tell me how well-behaved and well-mannered he was—wait, are we talking about *my* child? I certainly wished I saw more of that behaviour! I know many parents have had this experience. The teacher raves about your studious, compliant child and you wonder if they have mistaken which one is yours. Being on "best behaviour" can be exhausting for children, especially when the demands of the situation challenge their natural tendencies; this is why they may be able to hold it together in school, but then fall apart when they are back home "safe" with you, where they know they are loved even if they aren't their best selves.

But the other part is that people can perceive the same behaviour in different ways, as we discussed in chapter 2. My friend, who is a child psychologist, completed a series of temperament questionnaires about her young daughter and had her husband and nanny do the same. She said that she discovered they were all raising a different child! A child psychologist named Thomas Achenbach has been a leader in examining how different people perceive the same child's behaviour. In one study, he reviewed more than 250 samples with reports on child behaviour by multiple informants, including mothers, fathers, teachers, peers, mental health workers, and the children themselves. He found that reporters who saw the child in similar situations (e.g. co-parents) shared ratings of the child's behaviour more often (correlating on average about 0.6), than people who saw the children in different settings (who correlated on average only at 0.28). Children's reports of their own behaviour only correlated 0.22 with other people's reports of their behaviour! Overall, the findings clearly indicate that different people can perceive the same child's behaviour in very separate ways.

So, the first point of disagreement can be over partners' perceptions of their child's behaviour, and whether it presents a problem or not. But the next point of disagreement can involve how partners perceive the other's parenting. What this means is that you might perceive your parenting to be one way, but your partner—or your child—might experience it differently. You might think of yourself as a warm parent with clear boundaries and expectations, but your partner (or your child) might not see you that way.

Try this exercise with your partner: draw the parenting axes from the figure above (warmth/demandingness; low to high) on two sheets of paper. You and your partner each indicate with an X on your own sheet of paper where you think you fall, and where you think the other parent/partner falls, on the two dimensions. In this way, each co-parent/partner will rate him/herself and the other parent/partner. Once you are both done, compare your Xs. Do they match up? How close are you in your perceptions of each other's parenting?

Doing this exercise with my son's father was eye-opening. We had a lot of conflict surrounding our parenting styles when my son was young.

But when it came to rating ourselves, we both thought of ourselves as squarely within the Authoritative Parenting quadrant. Within the quadrant I rated myself as slightly higher on warmth and lower on demandingness, and he rated himself as slightly higher on demandingness and lower on warmth, but still—we both viewed ourselves as the "ideal" Authoritative parents.

But our views of each other didn't match up. I thought he fell into the Authoritarian parenting style, and he thought I fell into the Permissive parenting style. In other words, we agreed that I was higher on warmth and he was higher on demandingness, but we differed in the degree to which we perceived each other's balance of warmth and demandingness. He thought I was too warm without enough rules and boundaries (Permissive); I thought he was too strict and rule-bound without enough warmth (Authoritarian).

So who was right?

Naturally I was, since I have the Ph.D.

Kidding! Although if I am entirely honest, I definitely spent a long time thinking that I "objectively" had a more accurate perception of how best to parent. And if you're honest with yourself, you might find that you usually think your way is the "right" way too. We think that our way is best, because it's a reflection of how our brain works. It's what's right for us. And it's our reality.

This gets at the heart of why parenting is so hard—we have deeply rooted judgements attached to it based on the lens through which we see the world. Parenting in a vacuum would be much easier. In the real world, everyone involved in the process has a potentially different take on what constitutes love, boundaries, rewards, consequences, and more.

Getting on the Same Page

So what do you do when you and your partner's Xs are far apart? Use it as a starting point for conversation. Take turns asking each other to explain each of your perceptions of the partner's parenting.

What makes them think you are less warm? Or more demanding? Each partner should try to generate specific examples for the other partner that lead to their perception.

Why do they think it is important to have stricter (or fewer) rules? Why do they place more (or less) emphasis on flexibility?

When having these conversations, it is important to follow five steps so that your conversation is productive.

Listen to your partner's perspective. The goal of the conversation is *not* to try to convince them of the error of their ways, or to sway them to adopt your viewpoint; it is to try to understand where they are coming from. When your partner is sharing or providing examples, do not interrupt to tell them why they are interpreting things wrong. Your job is to *really* listen to the other person and try to understand their perspective. Frequently, when we have a conversation with someone whose views differ from our own, we are spending most of the time that they are talking thinking about all the reasons they are wrong, and formulating our rebuttal. Those skills might work in debate, but they aren't going to get you any closer to building a strong, unified co-parenting relationship. You may not agree with everything (or anything) they are saying, but you will come away with a deeper understanding of how they perceive the world. That's all you're trying to do initially: to learn about their perspective. You are not deciding or discussing whether you think it is right or wrong. You are just listening and learning.

Try to find common ground. This is where you start to work together. What do you agree on? Maybe you can both agree that having a warm relationship with your child is important; you just differ in what that means to each of you. Maybe you can agree that some degree of rules and boundaries is necessary, even if you differ in what those rules, and their enforcement, looks like. Maybe all you can agree on is that you don't like temper tantrums, or a particular behaviour that your child displays. Start with whatever common ground you can find.

List your differences. There is power in naming something. It takes some of the energy out of the proverbial elephant in the room. Use "I" statements as you are creating a list of places where you differ in your parenting styles. For example, do not say, "You never discipline Sally when she acts out"; say, "I think it's critical for children to have consequences to learn what we expect of them. I don't see you implementing consequences". As you are listing your differences, feel free to ask "why" questions to continue to learn more about their perspective. The key is to remember that neither partner gets to argue with the other's perspective here; you are just writing down the areas where you differ.

Come up with a plan for addressing your differences. Here's where the rubber meets the road. You now have a list of the things you have in common—your shared hopes or concerns about your child. And you have a list of your differences in how each of you is disposed to parent your child. Using the ideas from the previous chapters on creating Goodness of Fit for children with different temperamental styles, try to come up with a small number of actions that you can agree to implement. Maybe your partner is not ready to alter discipline strategies related to your child's Emotionality, but they are willing to try a When-Then plan to improve their Effortful Control. Make a list of the different recommended parenting strategies for your child's temperament, and work with your partner to identify which ones they are also on board with implementing. If they are strongly opposed to a certain strategy, table that for now and start with the ones you can agree on.

Evaluate and regroup. As a scientist and researcher, I hate to say this, but parenting is as much of an art as it is a science. Yes, we can use the research to guide us, but, try as we might, researchers can never fully take into account the myriad factors that impact any one child's outcome at a particular point in time. Children's behaviour is a product of a complex multitude of factors: their genetic predispositions across many dimensions, their home environments, their neighbourhoods, their cultures, their schools, other peers, siblings, the adults in their life, the environmental events they have experienced. Children are complex beings. And parenting is equally complex.

Parenting falls on a continuum, and is partly "in the eyes of the beholder", meaning that there are many ways to be a "good parent"—squarely inside the Authoritative quadrant, but differing in particular rules and strategies. In fact, the unique nature of each individual child *should* lead parents to move around within that quadrant, adopting different strategies for different children. The extension of "there is no one right way to parent" means that there can be different ways of implementing the strategies I have delineated in this book. Parenting is about trial and error.

Remembering the mantra "children are complex, parenting is complex" can help you work with your partner to come up with parenting strategies together. Keeping in mind that no one is objectively "right" can help you compromise to find strategies both of you can live with. Remember that nothing has to be forever. Agree on a strategy to try out, implement it, and see how it goes. This is where science is on your side. Even if you aren't thrilled with a parenting strategy that your partner wants to use, assuming it does not cause physical harm to your child, you can come up with a defined period of time to try it out, with a set plan to regroup and re-evaluate together how it is going at the end of the trial period. Be sure to allow enough time for your child to adapt to any new set of rules. Recall that children are likely to act out when rules change or anything new is introduced, so you should allow for at least a few weeks to get into a new routine and see how it goes. Then be willing to adjust and adapt as needed depending on the outcome.

Agree to Disagree

Understanding your partner's views on parenting does not mean that you have to agree with them. You may understand their perspective and where it comes from, but you still think your own way is "better". Rather than trying to bend your partner to your will, which can have the unintended effect of creating more tension in the home, sometimes the best path is to agree to disagree. Yes, it is ideal when parents can agree on their parenting strategy. But even when parents agree in principle, I have seen the most loving partners disagree about their parenting in practice. It can be hard for many of us to see our partner parent in ways that are not *exactly* in line with what we would do.

In reality, sometimes what works for one parent doesn't work for the other parent. Your partner may be trying to implement the same strategy, but because they come at it with a different disposition, it is perceived differently by the child. Children are smart. They quickly figure out that adults have different styles and ways of being. They learn, both consciously and unconsciously, how to adapt their behaviour to each of the adults in their life. This is actually an important life skill. So don't worry too much if you and your partner have somewhat different strategies with your child.

My ex-husband and I ultimately found that there were certain rules and strategies that we would consistently uphold across our households (my son split time between our homes), and there were certain things that one or the other of us implemented at our own house based on our own parenting styles. On the one hand, for example, I wanted more shared sticker charts and reward systems that would transfer across our households; he wanted firmer rules surrounding how we handled our picky eater. Ultimately, neither of us was willing to adopt the other's system; it didn't work for the other parent. On the other hand, when it came to homework and media use, we both felt strongly about having the same policies in place across our homes, and we were able to come up with a set of guidelines we both agreed on. In the early days, I worried a lot about the less-than-ideal (to my mind) lack of "full consistency" across our parenting team, but in the end, it turned out just fine. My son adapted and, ultimately, he ended up inadvertently driving our parenting styles to be far more similar than we originally had been at the beginning.

When your child is older, you can actually include them in the parenting styles exercise and ask them to indicate with Xs where they think each parent falls. You may find it to be eye-opening. But be prepared: your child's view will almost certainly differ from yours. If you do this exercise with them, be sure to follow the number 1 rule above: your objective in doing the exercise is to learn about their perception, *not* to tell them they are wrong.

This can be very hard. I recently did this exercise with my now-thirteen-year-old son. He rated me as lower on warmth than I perceived myself to be, and the reasons he gave were enlightening, but to my mind not particularly accurate or fair: "Remember that one time when I broke my arm and you didn't take me to the hospital?" It took every ounce of control not to say, "You have got to be kidding me! You cite that one time I was away on a business trip, and not the tons of times I was with you in the hospital and for doctor's appointments! I'm very high on warmth!"

OK, true confession, I might have actually said that. What I should have said was, "That's interesting that you see it that way. You know, I can't always be around to protect you from getting hurt. That's part of growing up. But what I can do is make sure that you are always loved and cared for so that when something happens, you know you will always be taken care of. That's why I think of myself as high on warmth."

The idea is to use the exercise as a means to share perspectives. But it doesn't mean you will always agree. So be forewarned. It may give you food for thought as a parent. For example, if you are aiming for an authoritative parenting style, but your child views you as authoritarian, might there be ways for you to allow more input from your child? Are there rules for which there might be some flexibility so that the child perceives some sharing in the decision-making process? Your perceived authoritarian style might reflect a family value surrounding the importance of respecting parents. That is an understandable value to want to impart to your child. But presumably you don't want a child who always complies with adults; you probably want your child to learn to think for themselves too. While an outspoken child may come across as questioning your rules, having conversations about parenting with your child can help you understand each other's perspective.

Note that "food for thought" does not mean that your child calls the shots on how you parent. I'm quite sure I would have loved for my parents to be more permissive when I was a teenager. I perceived their rules (I have a curfew?!) as authoritarian. But they were simply good parents who insisted on knowing where their teenager was, who I was with, and what I was doing. As a developmental psychologist (and parent of a teenager now), I appreciate the importance of parental monitoring in a way that I didn't when I was a teen. Remember, your child's brain is still under development, so their perceptions are likely to change across development.

There's one other piece to consider related to changes across time. Your child's temperament will play out differently at different developmental stages. This can create a different Goodness of Fit with different parents (or other adults) at different times as they are growing up. For example, low Effortful Control in a toddler could lead to a lot of commotion and broken household items. This may be very challenging for one parent who, for example, has designed a carefully curated house, while the other parent may not find it as upsetting. But low Effortful Control in a teenager could lead to high risk behaviours, such as alcohol use or other drug experimentation, and that may be far more challenging for the other parent to handle. So if you find that your temperament and your child's temperament grate against each other, or perhaps you envy that your child seems to be a much better "fit" with their other parent, know that this may change over time.

Setting Your Child Up for Success at School

Our children's temperaments influence the way they move through the world, and this extends to the school setting. Your child's genetic dispositions will have a big impact on their interactions at school, influencing their relationships with other children, the way they navigate the many demands of the school setting, and their relationships with their teachers. A child who is high on Extraversion may have no trouble making new friends in the classroom, whereas the Low Ex child may take longer to warm up to new peers. A High Em child may have trouble with transitions between activities during the school day. A Low Ef child may find it impossible to be in a classroom that involves a lot of stationary learning in one's seat. Just as the differences among our children's dispositions create unique challenges at home, children with different dispositions will have varied challenges in the school setting.

School brings many demands—one has to interface with other children, and learn what to do and what not to do: when it's OK to talk, and when you need to be quiet; when you have to stay in your seat, and when it's appropriate to move around. Individual differences in children's dispositions are obvious to anyone who has ever spent time in a classroom. There is the child who blurts out answers; the child who sits quietly; the child who can attentively focus on the teacher; the child who gets bored easily; the child who can stay seated at their desk; the child who is constantly bouncing in their chair; the child who easily makes lots of friends; and the child who keeps to him- or herself.

In the school setting, individual differences influence each child's success—both academically and socially—which impacts the feedback they receive from their peers and their teachers. This feedback, for good or bad, can further affect the way they see themselves and the way they experience people around them. Do they think of themselves as smart and likeable? Do they see other people as friendly and trustworthy?

Children's natural dispositions can influence their learning directly; for example, the Low Ef child who has trouble focusing on the teacher's lesson may have trouble learning the material. It can also impact their academic progress indirectly: for example, by influencing how disruptive they are in the classroom, which could impact their teacher's appraisal of them as a student. This, in turn, could affect whether the teacher chooses them for special academic programmes or honours.

There are many aspects of the school setting that teachers have no control over, such as the number of students in the classroom, the space that is available, and many routines in the daily school schedule. But there are other things that teachers can tweak, including how they arrange their classroom (who sits where), how they structure class activities (do they favour small group or large group activities), how transitions are handled (are there many or few), and how they manage behaviour. These differences in the classroom contribute to each child's Goodness of Fit at school. For example, a teacher who prefers large group activities and lesson plans involving the entire class may be a great fit for a highly extraverted child, who is more comfortable speaking up in front of their peers and being the centre of attention. The Low Ex child, however, may get lost in the crowd in these large group sessions. Instead, the Low Ex child may thrive when doing individual work or in small group activities. As another example, children who are low on Effortful Control may have trouble in a classroom where children are expected to stay and learn in their seats for much of the day, but they may do much better in a classroom with lots of activity where they are less constrained. In short, the "same" classroom is not the same for all children; it will be a better fit for some kids than others. Kids with temperaments that lead to problems in one classroom may thrive in another.

Of course, it's not only the classroom characteristics that differ, it's the teachers too. Teachers have their own natural dispositions, which influence the way they interact with and experience their students. Some teachers are more highly extraverted and full of energy, others are Low Ex and, sometimes, even withdrawn. Some will be higher on Emotionality—they may find the frustration of misbehaviour in the classroom more upsetting and challenging to deal with. Other teachers are more able to go with the flow and take it in stride. A child who repeatedly blurts out in class may be merely annoying to one teacher, but downright upsetting to another. Another teacher may find the child's enthusiastic outburst endearing.

Sometimes a teacher and a student have a natural Goodness of Fit, and sometimes they do not. For example, a Low Ex teacher may be particularly attuned to making sure her Low Ex students are not overlooked. But a High Ex teacher may wonder why Low Ex children don't speak up more in class and assume they are not as academically motivated or talented. Lived experience is important too. A teacher who grew up with a lot of rambunctious brothers may have no problem understanding and managing Low Ef boys, whereas another teacher may find their behaviour highly upsetting.

There's compelling evidence that the way teachers perceive their students matters: studies have found that children's temperament is correlated with teachers' assigned grades, and that this effect is much stronger when teachers have a more subjective role in grading (as opposed to, for example, multiple choice questions). Teachers have ideas about which students are most "teachable" or promising, and these preconceived notions impact their evaluations of children's academic performance.

Further, the interactions children have with their teachers affect their own appraisals of themselves as learners and as people. Teachers who give a lot of negative feedback can cause children to feel rejected, hurting their academic motivation and self-esteem. Conversely, teachers who embrace each child and work with them to develop their strengths and work on their challenges can have an important positive impact on students' academic self-concept, motivation, and accordingly, their academic achievement.

Great teachers understand that being aware of dispositional differences can help them; it can alleviate stress and enable them to reduce challenges in the classroom, just like recognising and adapting to kids' different dispositions can help parents at home. When there is a mismatch between temperament and the demands of their environment, children tend to misbehave—for some kids, the stressor may be a chaotic classroom; for other kids, it may be when the classroom is too structured. Some children won't react well to a teacher who calls on them in class to speak up in front of their peers; other kids need more individual recognition of their perseverance and effort. Just like with parents, if a teacher views a child's behaviour (failure to sit in their seat, refusal to speak up in class) as deliberate, rather than as an individual difference rooted in disposition, they are more likely to punish the child. Without understanding children's natural dispositions, they perceive the child as lacking the motivation to perform or behave, rather than lacking the skills.

So what can parents do about that? Teachers are often overworked and underpaid, as many parents more deeply appreciated during the COVID-19 pandemic of 2020, when parents were suddenly thrust into the role of homeschooling their children. While parents have the dispositions of their own children to contend with, teachers have an entire classroom of different dispositions to manage, and all the unique interactions among them. Further, the mix that they have to wrangle changes every year! On top of that, they are responsible for teaching the children academic material, while attending to their individual emotional and behavioural development. Teachers have hard jobs!

You know your child better than anyone, and often teachers will appreciate your insight. If you think that your child may have particular challenges in the school setting, don't be afraid to talk to the teacher about it. It's best if you can have these conversations proactively, before problems start to arise. Frame it in the context of your child's natural disposition, to make teachers aware of how they may see it play out in the classroom setting. I try to do this at the start of the school year, in whatever forum is most appropriate for the school. For example, some schools have "open hours" to meet the teacher before the start of school, others have parent–teacher conferences at the start of the year. Some schools send home forms asking parents if there is "anything they should know" about your child; use this opportunity to let you teacher know about temperamental characteristics that may affect your child's behaviour or performance in the school setting. If your school doesn't have any options where you will have time to have a one-on-one conversation with the teacher, you can always send them an email or give them a call, depending on your child's teacher's preferred method of communication.

Here are some examples of how you might approach this kind of conversation:

> *"Hi Mr/Mrs Teacher, my daughter, Taylor, is in your class this year. Taylor is naturally introverted, so I just wanted to give you a heads-up that sometimes she needs encouragement to speak up in class. She does really well in small group settings, but is often intimidated to raise her hand in front of the whole class."*

> *"James is full of energy! We're still working with him on self-control, and sometimes he has trouble holding back from blurting out or interrupting. We've found that when he seems to be having trouble restraining himself, it can help if there is something active he can do to refocus. For example, his teacher last year would give him an errand to run to the school office, or papers to sort in the back of the classroom."*

> *"Brianna is naturally a really emotional child. She can have trouble when she gets frustrated. Some things we've found that help her calm down at home are . . ."*

In these conversations, you are helping the teacher understand your child's natural tendencies, and, where possible, providing ideas for solutions to address challenges that you are using at home or that have worked in the past. Note that you are not telling the teacher what to do, nor can you expect that the teacher will, for example, put in place the same behaviour programme that you are implementing at home, or that another teacher used last year. Teachers, like most of us, have lots of demands placed upon them, and they will respond much better to you (and by extension, to your child) when you frame the conversation as an effort to provide them with helpful information to understand and work with your child, rather than as an attempt to tell them how to run their classroom.

Some parents express concern that having these conversations up front will colour the teacher's impression of their child. The reality is that your child's teacher is going to figure out their disposition—for good and bad—whether you talk to them about it or not. It is always better to be proactive rather than reactive. Certain dispositions can create challenges in the school setting, but in many cases, modifications that are under the teacher's control can help alleviate some of those challenges. By talking to the teacher beforehand, you can help them put systems in place to support your child and their growth, rather than ending up in a situation that causes problems for all.

Think through what aspects of your child's tendencies might lead to challenges in school: Does your child have trouble with transitions? Do they find it challenging to sit quietly? Does your child get overstimulated? Do they have trouble with large groups? Proactively talking with your child's teacher about your child's disposition and areas where they may have difficulty, and working together on ways to handle or minimise challenges, can help set your child up for success in school. At the end of the day, both teachers and parents have the common goal of wanting the child to succeed. Here are some common challenges associated with different dispositional traits at school to help guide you as you consider your own child:

- High Ex children, who tend to enjoy being around other children and engaging in new activities, often feel right at home in the school setting. When coupled with low Effortful Control, however, they may have trouble refraining from blurting out answers or talking to peers during class time. You can work with your High Ex, Low Ef child to build their self-control skills, and discuss the need to apply those strategies when they are in school as well as at home.

- Low Ex children can be overlooked in the school setting, especially in large classrooms, where they are less likely to speak up, especially with more highly extraverted children in the classroom. If teachers are not aware of children's more quiet nature, they may perceive them as less motivated or less intelligent because they participate less actively in group settings. Low Ex children's preference for a smaller number of close friends can create challenges when they change classrooms each year and may be separated.

- Children low in Effortful Control can have difficulties at school because there are many tasks that require exerting self-control—sitting at one's desk quietly, focusing on schoolwork, not talking to friends, not interrupting the teacher. Working with your child on self-control strategies can also help them in the school setting.

- High Emotionality can lead to a number of challenges at school. High Em children by definition have trouble with distress, frustration, or fear, and being in school can create a lot of scenarios that lead to those feelings! Your High Em child's triggers will help you think through the particular scenarios that may present challenges for your child. For example, your High Em child may be more likely to get distressed by demands to transition between activities, or requirements to engage in novel activities that are out of their comfort zone, such as a school trip or the school play.

- An important extra word here on High Em children: sometimes their misbehaviour at home can be related to a school-related stressor, even if it's not immediately obvious.

When my son was in early primary school, we'd have a great morning together, but just as we were walking to the car to head to school he would suddenly throw down his school bag, storm back into the house, and declare that he wasn't going to school. Dumbfounded, I'd think, "What the heck?" Naturally, this seemed to happen most frequently when I had to head to an important work meeting directly after school drop-off. Needless to say, in my frustration and confusion (and hurry), I was not my best parenting self. This is the problem with being reactive instead of proactive.

Over time, I discovered that these emotional outbursts were a result of his remembering something school-related that he was anxious about as we headed to the car. There were a number of things that triggered his distress response: he would realise that he had forgotten to do a homework assignment, or that they were going to be working on a project he was having trouble with. Or—worst of all for a fear-prone High Em, Low Ex child—it was school play practice day. I had many conversations with his teachers over the years about the dreaded school play and the havoc it wreaked at our house. Needless to say, I could not have been more proud (and relieved) to see my miserable-looking Rock (yes, one year he was cast as a rock in the school play) onstage on performance day. You have to meet your children where they are—and sometimes that means being delighted to see your child perform as the Rock, rather than in the lead role.

Most teachers are happy to have engaged parents who are trying to help them set their child up for success. Most, but not all. Just like with co-parents, grandparents, and other adults, there are some teachers who are set in their ways, have strong opinions about managing children's behaviour, and are unwilling to modify their style to adapt flexibly to different children. Sadly, some teachers are not interested in being active partners with parents. When you encounter one of those teachers, and when there is also clearly not a strong Goodness of Fit (either for you or your child!), you can still work with your child at home on strategies to manage their challenges at school. Remember, this too shall pass and your child will have a new teacher next year.

It Takes a Village

There will be many adults who play a role in your child's life as they grow up: coaches, grandparents, neighbours, activity leaders. Your child's Goodness of Fit with each of them will influence their development in ways that are not entirely predictable. As a parent, you obviously can't expect everyone to adapt to your child, or to adopt the parenting style that you have found to work best for your child. So how do you decide when it is worth having a conversation about your child's disposition? This is a bigger concern for parents of children whose natural tendencies cause challenges across a variety of settings. There's no clear right answer (I hate that!). The rule of thumb that I use is that if it is a person who is going to be spending a lot of time with my child *and* I think it likely that the setting in which they interact with my child will create dispositional challenges, I will proactively have the conversation. If their interactions with my child are more limited, and the situation is one in which I don't think there is a high probability of problems (famous last words), then I usually see how it goes and only address issues if and when they arise. Grandparents coming to watch my children for a week when my husband and I go on holiday: proactive conversation. Grandparents who visit once a year for a quick trip: hope for the best. The nanny who watches my child after school gets a long proactive talk (usually before we make a hiring decision); the occasional babysitter may just get a few quick instructions about the bedtime routine. As adults, we make decisions all the time about how much information is necessary to provide to any given individual at any given time (my best friend gets a full account of last night's disagreement with my husband, the air-conditioning repair man does not); conversations about your children's dispositions are no different.

Takeaways

- Parents tend to vary along two key dimensions: warmth and demandingness.

- The way we view parenting is a reflection of our own unique, genetically influenced temperamental styles. This is true of the way our children view our parenting, the way we view ourselves as parents, the way we view our partner's parenting, and the way our partners view our parenting.

- It is important for co-parents to make an effort to understand each other's perspective on parenting.

- Each parent's disposition will interact with the child's disposition in different ways, which is why the strategies one person adopts may not always work for the other.

- Children's temperamental characteristics will impact their Goodness of Fit at school.

- Talking with your child's teacher about their natural tendencies can help you create a partnership to address potential challenges and help your child succeed academically.

CHAPTER 8

When to Worry, What to Do

Parents frequently ask me, "How do I know if my child has a disorder?"

When does High Emotionality tip over to become anxiety? How much impulsivity is too much? Are my child's extreme temper tantrums normal? Does my child have low self-control, or ADHD? These are questions that many parents struggle with.

Even with a Ph.D. in clinical psychology, I am no exception. I wrestled with these issues with my own son. It can be hard to tell what's "within normal range", especially because unless you have a job that puts you around lots of children (e.g. you're a teacher or a day-care provider), generally you have a small sample size of reference points to work from. What's "normal" when it comes to kids anyway? My son slept on pillows on the ground next to his perfectly comfortable bed *for a year*. When I was a child, I refused to eat anything other than bananas for months. It's hard to figure out what's "normal" in children.

A big reason it is so difficult to know whether a behaviour is within normal range or clinically concerning is that there is no clear answer. Human behaviour falls on a bell-shaped continuum, with some people being lower on any given trait, lots of us in the middle, and some individuals at the higher end. In statistics we call this pattern of variability a *normal distribution.* So, by definition, it's normal for some people to be high on a trait. Our genetic predispositions impact where we fall on that continuum. When we define clinical disorders, such as anxiety, depression, or attention-deficit hyperactivity disorder (ADHD), we are essentially drawing an arbitrary line on that curve and saying that people above a certain level of worry, sadness, or impulsivity exceed a threshold that we consider problematic. But there is no clear line between normal behavioural variation and behavioural disorders. There is no litmus test or biomarker to indicate whether a child has a disorder or not.

Even the experts don't have a very precise way of defining when a behaviour crosses the line to a disorder. Behavioural disorders are diagnosed based on symptom checklists created by committees of psychiatrists and psychologists, which in turn are based on their clinical judgement and expertise. In the United States, diagnoses are made based on the *Diagnostic and Statistical Manual of Mental Disorders (DSM-5)*, which is published by the American Psychiatric Association and is currently in its fifth edition. In the UK, however, clinicians use the WHO's International Classification of Diseases (ICD-10) system to diagnose mental disorders. How disorders are defined changes with every new edition of both the DSM and ICD, sometimes just a little and sometimes drastically (homosexuality was once classified as a disorder). Every ten to fifteen years, for instance, the DSM is revised; it's a process that involves hundreds of researchers and clinicians, and takes years of discussion and heated debate. The World Health Organization's *International Statistical Classification of Diseases and Related Health Problems* (ICD) is currently in the process of releasing it *eleventh* version, and follows a similar process.

That is to say, behavioural disorders are defined in imprecise and ever-changing ways. What we do know is that behavioural and emotional challenges are extremely common in children. Estimates vary, but approximately one in five children meet criteria for a diagnosable mental health disorder. A recent report from the US National Academies of Sciences, Engineering, and Medicine states that the most common disorders in children are anxiety, affecting about 30 per cent of children between the ages of six and seventeen years. According to NHS 24 figures, in the UK between 5 and 19 per cent of all children and adolescents suffer from anxiety disorders. behavioural disorders, such as attention-deficit hyperactivity disorder (ADHD) or oppositional defiant disorder (ODD), affecting about 20 per cent of children in the US (in the UK those numbers are between 3 and 5 per cent); and depression, affecting about 15 per cent of children in the US (about 10 per cent of children in the UK suffer from depression according to the Mental Health Foundation). Children who meet criteria for these disorders are children whose fears, frustrations, or impulsivity are sufficiently high that they are causing significant problems in their lives.

Psychologists talk about behavioural and emotional problems in children as falling along two dimensions, called *internalising* and *externalising*. These terms reflect how a child channels their emotional challenges: internally or externally. *Internalising* refers to problems that children experience on the inside, such as anxiety or depression. *Externalising* refers to problems that children manifest externally, meaning that children act out. Attention-deficit hyperactivity and oppositional defiant disorder are examples of externalising disorders. The terms *internalising* and *externalising* remind us that these behaviours are continuums, with disorders representing the upper end of human behavioural variation, rather than separate "things" that people inherit. No one inherits a mental health disorder; we simply inherit different ways of brain functioning, some of which are more likely to create challenges at the extreme.

High Em children are more at risk of both internalising and externalising disorders, since by definition they have a heightened predisposition towards fear and frustration. Some High Em children are more inclined to internalise; they turn their fears and upset inward, resulting in elevated rates of anxiety or depression. For other High Em children, their natural tendency to be easily frustrated may turn outwards, leading to hitting, throwing things, or other explosive behaviour. If these behaviours are severe enough, they may meet criteria for the externalising disorder called *oppositional defiant disorder* (ODD). Children who have low Effortful Control by definition have trouble controlling their impulsive tendencies; they are at elevated risk for externalising disorders, in particular ADHD. As they get older, they are also more at risk for substance use disorders.

I'm going to walk you through the most common internalising and externalising disorders in children, to help you better understand the symptoms associated with each. As we're stepping through different diagnoses, remember that meeting criteria for a mental health disorder doesn't mean that there is something "wrong" with your child; it just means that your child inherited a brain that is wired in a more extreme way. They are on the upper end of traits that vary continuously across the population. Their unique genetic constitution makes it more difficult for them to function in their environment. That means they may need some extra help—more intense behavioural interventions to tackle their challenges or, in some cases, medication to help their brains get to a level of functioning that is less extreme, allowing them to operate better in their day-to-day lives.

Another thing to keep in mind as we are reviewing various symptoms is that children diagnosed with one mental health challenge are at greater risk of being diagnosed with additional disorders. We call this *comorbidity*, and it refers to the fact that many behavioural and emotional challenges cluster together, and sometimes can be hard to separate. In general, children with an internalising problem (e.g. anxiety) are more at risk for other internalising problems (e.g. depression). Similarly, children diagnosed with one externalising disorder (e.g. ODD) are more at risk for other externalising disorders (e.g. ADHD). This is because internalising disorders share genetic influences, meaning that there are common genes that give rise to multiple types of internalising. A parallel situation is true of externalising disorders: there are genes that can elevate risk for a variety of externalising problems.

Behavioural challenges can also create cascades, in that one area of difficulty can lead to other problems. For example, if a child's anxiety interferes with their ability to make friends, that may cause loneliness, which could bring on depression. Conversely, another child's anxiety may cause them to experience intense frustration and anger, which could lead to defiant and oppositional behaviour. This is why it's important to identify and seek help for behavioural challenges early.

Internalising Disorders—Challenges Experienced Inside

Anxiety

Anxiety is the most commonly diagnosed mental health problem, both in children and adults. The good news is that anxiety disorders are highly treatable; however, many people with anxiety never get treatment. Often this is because, despite the many ways that anxiety interferes with one's life, many people don't realise that it doesn't have to be that way. It's all they've ever known, so, sadly, they assume it's just their lot in life to live with anxiety. Accordingly, we're going to discuss anxiety at some length, so you know what signs to look for in your child.

People with anxiety experience worry and fear at such a high level that it interferes with their day-to-day lives. Some people erroneously believe that children with anxiety will "grow out of it" or just need to "toughen up". Anxiety, however, isn't a problem that resolves on its own. Instead, it tends to worsen over time. Accordingly, the earlier you seek help, the sooner your child can learn skills to manage their fears.

If you're not someone who experiences clinical-level anxiety, it can be difficult to understand why children with anxiety can't just "get over it". That's because all of us have some experience with anxiety. We may feel nervous or fearful when we are trying something new, or uncertain about how something will turn out. It's normal to feel a bit anxious before you go onstage for a performance or give a speech in front of an audience. How much anxiety you experience in various situations will be a product of your genetic make-up (how naturally prone you are towards fear and worry) and your life experiences. On the one hand, if you've given dozens of talks, you will probably feel less anxious than you did for the first one. On the other hand, if the last time you gave a talk it didn't go well, then you may feel more nervous the next time. These are normal human experiences.

It may seem hard to believe, but some degree of anxiety is actually a good thing—it's what makes us study for an exam or practise for a play, out of fear of doing poorly. Fear is evolutionarily adaptive. Being cautious helps human beings stay alive. If early humans had no fear, they would have been eaten by lions and tigers and bears (oh my!). Our ability to recognise the possibility of bad things happening is what keeps us safe. Behavioural traits that help keep us alive get passed down to future generations, which is why human beings continue to have some level of fear and worry.

Anxious children, however, have brains that err too much on the side of worry. The part of the brain that processes fear and perceived threat, called the *amygdala*, is overactive; this leads anxious children to see potential danger everywhere. Their brains are on high alert for possible negative outcomes, and they overestimate the possibility that bad things may happen. So a child with anxiety may look at the sea and think, "Danger! Sharks!" Usually the prefrontal cortex, which you'll recall from chapter 6 is the part of the brain that allows for cool, rational response, helps put this fear response in context; it reminds us that shark attacks are very rare, and there are lifeguards who are on the lookout. But in a child with anxiety, their prefrontal cortex is no match for their overactive amygdala. Their amygdala just keeps screaming, "DANGER! SHARKS!" and drowns out everything else. In this way, their anxiety goes unchecked and starts interfering with their functioning instead of just keeping them safe.

Anxiety is not technically a single thing; there are a whole class of anxiety disorders, including:

Generalised anxiety disorder–characterised by excessive worry about many things, ranging from school to friends to sports.

Specific phobias–characterised by intense, irrational fear of a particular object or situation (for example, fear of dogs or flying).

Social anxiety disorder–characterised by intense fear of social situations and activities.

Obsessive-compulsive disorder (OCD)–characterised by unwanted intrusive thoughts (obsessions) and a compelling need to complete a ritualised behaviour (for example, a series of tapping) in an effort to alleviate the resulting anxiety.

Panic disorder–characterised by sudden attacks of overwhelming fear, often accompanied by physiological symptoms such as elevated heart rate and shortness of breath.

Post-traumatic stress disorder (PTSD)–characterised by intense fear or anxiety brought on by experiencing or witnessing a traumatic event.

The specific symptoms vary for each type of anxiety disorder, which is why it is important to talk to a professional who can help determine a diagnosis and formulate a treatment plan accordingly. But here are some general signs to look for which may indicate that your child suffers from an anxiety disorder:

- Does your child seem to excessively worry about a lot of things, in a way that seems out of proportion?

- Do they worry more days than not? Is their worry starting to dominate your daily routine or activities?

- Is it hard for your child to control their worry? Do your efforts to try to reason with them and put their worry in context seem to have no impact on their worrying?

- Is their worry negatively impacting their ability to function—to go to school, to interact with friends? Is it interfering with family routines and activities?

- Does your child complain of headaches or stomach aches, or regularly tell you that they don't feel well when it is time to go to school or other outings?

- Does your child have challenges sleeping, or frequent nightmares?

- Is your child excessively concerned that others are upset with them, or worried about what others think about them?

- Is your child refusing to participate in school or sports activities?

- Is your child easily distressed or angered by stressful situations?

- Do you spend an excessive amount of time consoling your child about their distress over ordinary situations?

- Does your child express constant "what if" worries that are not ameliorated by talking through them together?

If the answer to one or more of the above questions is yes, consider seeking professional help.

One final thing to keep in mind is that some children, particularly boys, respond to their anxiety by acting out and misbehaving. This can be confusing because it blurs the line between internalising (what they're experiencing internally) and externalising behaviour (their acting out). Instead of saying, "I'm really nervous to go to school", they will instead throw down their books as you're walking to the bus and defiantly declare, "I'm not going to school and you can't make me!". Children who respond to underlying anxiety with irritability or temper tantrums may end up evoking parental consequences and anger, rather than empathy. It can take longer to realise that this behaviour is a reflection of anxiety. If you find that your child is having outbursts that coincide with social situations (going to school, participating in sports or camps, the dreaded school play), then the underlying cause of the behaviour may actually be anxiety.

Mind UK provides useful information and support for anxiety, depression and other mental health issues for all ages (mind.org.uk). The Anxiety and Depression Association of America (adaa.org) has wonderful resources and is a great place to learn more about anxiety.

Depression

Everyone feels sad or down sometimes, but individuals with depressive disorders have persistent sadness that interferes with their daily lives. Similar to anxiety, there are actually a number of depressive disorders, but when people talk about depression, they are usually referring to major depressive disorder (MDD). MDD involves a period of depression lasting more than two weeks. Depression is less common than anxiety disorders in young children, which is why we will cover it more briefly. Many children who have anxiety disorders, however, go on to develop depression later—often in their teens. Depression is more common in girls than in boys.

Here are some indicators that your child may be suffering from depression:

- Is your child frequently sad or tearful, or cries a lot?
- Has your child lost interest in activities that they used to enjoy?
- Is your child withdrawing from social activities or friends?

- Is your child having difficulty concentrating?
- Does your child express hopelessness?
- Does your child seem to have low self-esteem or a very harsh assessment of themselves (e.g. I'm no good, I'll never make friends, I'm ugly)?
- Has your child had a major change in their eating or sleeping patterns?
- Does your child talk about wanting to die?
- Does your child have increased irritability or temper tantrums?
- Does your child have decreased energy?
- Does your child report many aches or pains without an obvious cause?

You'll note that some of the symptoms of depression overlap with indicators of anxiety—for example, heightened irritability, problems sleeping, and reporting headaches or stomach aches. This again reflects the fact that depression and anxiety, though technically diagnosed as separate disorders, actually have shared underlying genetic influences. Individuals inherit a general predisposition towards internalising—a disposition towards turning strong emotions such as fear, worry, or distress inwards. In some people this disposition shows up more as anxiety, and in other people it manifests as depression. It can also show up differently in the same person over time—as anxiety at one point in development, and depression at another. This is why it is so important to get help early.

Cognitive behavioural therapy (CBT) is a well-established, scientifically backed treatment for anxiety and depression (as well as other psychological conditions) that has been proven effective. It helps individuals recognise their thinking patterns, learn to control negative thinking and worry, and modify their behavioural responses. In this way, individuals gain an understanding of how their brain is naturally programmed, and build skills (and accordingly, new brain connections) that enable better coping. For example, instead of allowing their brain to scream "DANGER! SHARKS!" and throw them into a panic, individuals learn to recognise their overactive worry brain (or negative thinking brain in the case of depression), and to build new, more rational and adaptive responses by strengthening prefrontal cortex responses to help them counteract that natural tendency.

Externalising Disorders—Challenges Channelled Outwards

Oppositional Defiant Disorder (ODD)

ODD is one of the most commonly diagnosed behavioural disorders in children. Children with ODD tend to have high Emotionality and low Effortful Control. They have trouble managing their frustrations and anger, and difficulty controlling themselves in response to their strong feelings. ODD is defined by a pattern of negative, hostile behaviour that lasts at least six months. There's nothing magical about six months, but the idea is to ensure that the diagnosis is only made when there are *persistent* behavioural problems, not just passing defiant behaviour in children (because most parents experience at least some of that). ODD is considered present if a child meets at least four of the following criteria:

- Does your child often lose their temper?
- Is your child often angry and resentful?
- Does your child often argue with adults?
- Does your child frequently defy or refuse to comply with adults' requests or rules?
- Does your child intentionally annoy other people?
- Does your child frequently blame others for their mistakes?
- Is your child often spiteful or vindictive?

All children misbehave sometimes. ODD is diagnosed when the *duration* and *degree* of the challenging behaviour is greater than is typically observed for the child's age and developmental stage. Again, this doesn't mean there is anything "wrong" with the child (though parents frightened by their child's outbursts may worry this is the case); it just means the child is high on Emotionality and doesn't yet have the ability to manage it.

Treatments for ODD involve an intense regimen of the strategies we discussed for High Em children in chapter 5, and include working with parents so that they understand their child is lacking skills, not just trying to be manipulative or defiant; recognising triggers; and building on collaborative problem-solving strategies. Children diagnosed with ODD are at elevated risk for ADHD, due to the fact that high impulsivity elevates risk for multiple externalising outcomes. Children with ODD also have higher rates of subsequently developing anxiety or depression, likely due to the negative feedback loops that result when children act out in extreme ways; their behaviour may lead them to have challenges with peers, at home, and at school, causing them to internalise feelings of isolation or despair, which could lead to anxiety or depression. Accordingly, it is important to get help early.

Attention-Deficit Hyperactivity Disorder (ADHD)

ADHD is often described as a disorder of behavioural undercontrol, or behavioural disinhibition. In short, this means that children with ADHD have trouble controlling their impulses. Boys are more likely to meet criteria for ADHD than girls are. By definition, children with ADHD are low on Effortful Control; their brains are wired differently, in the ways we discussed in chapter 6. Children with ADHD have more trouble staying focused on tasks that they find boring; they tend to act before they think through the consequences; and they are often fidgety, active, and restless, more so than other children their age. Many children with ADHD have challenges with attention *and* impulsivity, but it is also possible to have problems predominantly with inattention *or* hyperactivity (rather than both).

Here are common signs of problems with inattention (diagnosis requires six or more from the list):

- Does your child fail to pay close attention to details or make careless mistakes?
- Does your child often have trouble keeping their attention focused on tasks or play activities?
- Does your child frequently not listen when spoken to directly?
- Does your child fail to finish schoolwork or chores?
- Does your child have trouble organising tasks or activities?
- Does your child avoid or dislike tasks that require sustained mental attention over a long period of time (like schoolwork)?
- Does your child often lose things necessary for tasks and activities (e.g. school materials, pencils, books, tools, wallets, keys, paperwork, eyeglasses, mobile phones)?
- Is your child often easily distracted?
- Is your child often forgetful in daily activities?

Listed below are symptoms of hyperactivity-impulsivity. At least six symptoms must be present for at least six months, and the symptoms must be disruptive and inappropriate for the child's developmental stage, for a diagnosis to be made:

- Does your child often fidget or tap their hands or feet, or squirm in their seat?
- Does your child often leave their seat in situations when remaining seated is expected?
- Does your child often run about or climb in situations where it is not appropriate?

- Is your child often unable to play or take part in leisure activities quietly?
- Is your child often "on the go," acting as if "driven by a motor"?
- Does your child often talk excessively?
- Does your child often blurt out an answer before a question has been completed?
- Does your child often have trouble waiting their turn?
- Does your child often interrupt or intrude on others (e.g. butts into conversations or games)?

In addition to meeting the above behavioural criteria, for a diagnosis of ADHD to be made, the behaviours must be present in two or more settings (e.g. both at home and school, or with parents as well as other caregivers). In addition, the symptoms have to be interfering with the child's functioning—for example, by causing problems at home or at school or with friends.

Disorder versus Temperament

As you were reading through the list of symptoms for each of the common childhood disorders, you likely recognised that they overlapped with the behaviours that we discussed in the context of different genetically influenced temperamental characteristics. For example, being highly active and talking excessively are common in High Ex children, but they are also criteria for ADHD. Being easily frustrated or quick to temper is indicative of high Emotionality, but it is also a symptom of ODD. Similarly, being fearful or irritable is a characteristic found in High Em children, but it is also among the symptoms listed for internalising disorders. Low Ef children have trouble with self-control, which is also a core feature of ADHD.

This may lead you to wonder, when is it temperament and when is it a disorder? If you're puzzling over this question, you have simply stumbled upon the reality that there is nothing sacred about clinical disorders. Children who are at the upper end of behavioural traits are by definition more extreme, which can lead them to have challenges in environments designed for the "average" person. Clinical disorders simply represent behaviour patterns that have been identified as causing challenges. Accordingly, if you are worried about your child because their behaviour is causing problems, I encourage you *not* to spend time wondering if they meet criteria for a disorder—remember, that's an arbitrary and imprecise threshold. Instead, go ahead and talk to a doctor or therapist any time you are concerned about your child's behaviour.

I have seen parents agonise over whether to seek help for their children's behavioural challenges. It doesn't have to be that hard. As parents, we make judgement calls about when to take our children to see a professional all the time. We do it every time they have a cough or a cut. We see symptoms like a sore throat or fever, and we decide when it is serious enough to merit a visit to the doctor for further investigation, and when to treat it with chicken soup and extra love at home. We aren't responsible for diagnosing them before we go to the doctor (although we might have guesses as to what's wrong); we just know something is wrong and we seek professional help.

Similarly, when it comes to our children's mental health, we can follow a parallel logic. We decide when, for example, a period of heightened fear will pass, and when it merits a call to a psychologist. Every temper tantrum doesn't trigger an appointment with a therapist, but a sustained pattern of frightening outbursts might warrant further examination. The lists of symptoms for common behavioural and emotional disorders can help you recognise potential areas of concern, but even these don't offer clear answers: they require behaviours to be present "often" or "frequently" or "a lot", which is a judgement call.

Accordingly, *the best rule of thumb to use in deciding whether to seek professional help is whether the behaviour is causing impairment.* Is your child's behaviour interfering with their relationship with you, with their peers, or with their teachers? Is your child repeatedly getting into trouble at school? Have they been kicked out of multiple playgroups? Are you trying your best to implement the strategies discussed in this book (and possibly others) and it doesn't feel like it's working? If your answer to any of those questions is yes, go ahead and reach out for extra help.

Another thing to take into account is whether your child has had a change in behaviour. If your child is normally a happy High Ex child, but suddenly starts spending a lot of time in their room, doesn't want to see their friends, or engage in activities that they used to love, then it is worth digging deeper to try to figure out what is going on. If the pattern of unusual behaviour persists (a general guideline is a month or more), then you want to consider seeking help.

One final note: if your child is displaying any signs that they may be a danger to themselves or others, seek help immediately. That doesn't mean that if your child makes a melodramatic comment ("If I don't make the team, I just want to die"), you have to speed-dial a psychiatrist. Use your parental intuition: if the threat to themselves or others feels real, then reach out.

How to Get Help

"That may be well and good", you think, "but where do I start if I want to get help for my child?" I wish that question had an easy answer, but unfortunately there is a lot of variability in the quality of therapists. You can't just open the phone book and call any therapist. Simply having a licence to practise doesn't guarantee that individual will provide the most effective treatment for your child. The lack of quality control in psychiatry and psychology is probably an artefact of the stigma that has surrounded mental health conditions—the belief that they are not "real" disorders in the way that other medical conditions are. Our understanding of mental health challenges, however, has come a long way. We now know that mental health disorders are genetically influenced, just like other biomedical disorders, and we also have evidence-based treatments that work. You want to make sure that's what your child gets.

I've compiled a list of resources to help you get started. It is by no means exhaustive, but it represents some of my go-to places for information that I know are grounded in the science. In the UK, you might start your search for help at your GP practice.

- The Institute of Mental Health (institutemh.org.uk)—seeks to help transform our understanding and treatment of mental illness.

- Young Minds (youngminds.org.uk)— the UK's leading charity fighting for children and young people's mental health.

- Royal College of Psychiatrists (rcpsych.ac.uk)—the professional and educational body for psychiatrists in the UK. It also provides information to the general public on common mental health issues and treatments.

- British Association for Behavioural and Cognitive Psychotherapies (www.babcp.com)—its website has extensive resources on CBT.

The reality is that you have to be an educated consumer when shopping for a mental health professional; even in the UK where the NHS provides mental health treatment free at the point of delivery. You have to do your homework. Unfortunately, you can't tell if someone will be a good therapist (meaning one who is delivering scientifically supported treatments) by how nice the waiting room is, or whether you get a good feeling at the practice. You need to ask questions of someone you are considering as a potential therapist. You want to ask the therapist:

- What treatment do you recommend?
- Is there scientific evidence to support this treatment?

- Are there other treatment options?
- Why do you use your preferred treatment over others?

Your first priority is to find someone who delivers scientifically supported interventions; however, this person is also someone with whom you're going to be developing a close working relationship. Accordingly, it's also appropriate to take into account your reaction to the clinician. You need to feel like you have a good rapport with the therapist—there's actually evidence that this plays a role in whether therapy is perceived to work! But keep in mind that who clicks for you will not necessarily click for your child; there was a particular therapist who I loved, but my child thought she was too much like me (!), so for him, it felt like he was getting a double dose of "mum tips".

Why Wait?
The Case for Seeking Help Sooner Rather Than Later

Here's the bottom line: if you're wondering if you should seek help—go ahead and do it! Maybe you're waiting to see if the behaviour gets better on its own, or if you can find ways of managing it. That's a normal first course of action, but if you find that reading books and trying to implement behavioural strategies on your own isn't working, then don't hesitate to seek additional help from a professional. Remember that the earlier you get help for your child, the sooner they can start learning skills to manage their challenges.

Some parents worry they will be judged. They are nervous about seeing a psychologist or psychiatrist. Here's the thing—therapists love working with people! They see lots of people whose children are struggling. They don't think there is anything wrong with people who seek help—they also love helping people! Therapists are trained to create a comfortable environment. The people I know who are most likely to seek professional help are other mental health professionals—we know that raising children is hard and we can all use extra help, especially from other people who have expertise in the science of child behaviour.

Another reason parents wait is because they have concerns that their child will be labelled. They don't want their child diagnosed with ADHD or an anxiety disorder (for example). They worry about the stigma that may surround a diagnosis. In my experience, most therapists are less concerned with making a diagnosis than they are with helping your family and your child in their struggles. Often it's the parents who are more worried about whether their child "has" a disorder. Most clinicians are well aware of the problems associated with clinical diagnoses. They recognise that children's behavioural challenges don't fit neatly into all-or-nothing boxes. In the US diagnoses are made primarily to help with health insurance, record keeping, and billing for treatment; fortunately, this is not the case in the UK where treatment is free at the point of delivery, which is why seeking help from your GP might be a good place to start.. Most clinicians avoid making diagnoses of children under five.

You want to weigh your concern about your child receiving a diagnosis against the harm of leaving behavioural and emotional challenges untreated. Anxiety, depression, ODD, ADHD, and other behavioural and emotional challenges can have severe adverse consequences when they are not addressed, affecting children's relationships with their parents, their ability to make friends, and their performance in school. These challenges can then further exacerbate problems, as children become increasingly despondent about their place in the world. Getting help for your child can help break these negative cycles and give them the skills they need to develop closer friendships, do better in school, and importantly, develop a better relationship with you, their parent.

For some children (and adults), receiving a diagnosis actually helps validate that what they are experiencing is "real". It helps them understand that many people struggle with the same challenges. It allows affected individuals and families to recognise that they are not alone, and to realise that there are treatments that can make things better. For many, a diagnosis actually brings hope, especially when approached with the growth mindset that we discussed in chapter 3.

Another concern for some parents is the potential cost associated with seeking help from a mental health professional. Help within the NHS structure in the UK is free, but if seeking private care or therapies, then the cost may be a issue. Cost and payment options are things you should discuss when talking with potential therapists. Some practices have sliding fee scales, and some private practices even do some pro bono work. If cost is a consideration, be up front with the therapist when inquiring about their services. If that individual or practice cannot accommodate your financial situation, they may be able to suggest other professionals that have more economical or flexible payment options.

The reality is that *all of us* can use help with parenting. For some of us, reading books and talking to friends is enough. But parents whose children have temperaments that are more challenging shouldn't hesitate to seek additional help, especially when those dispositions are interfering with their child's life or family functioning. Finding a professional who can partner with you to help implement science-based strategies to strengthen your child's lagging skills can be a much-needed lifeline.

Takeaways

- Behavioural and emotional challenges are very common in children, with anxiety and behavioural disorders (oppositional defiant disorder, ADHD) being the most common, followed by depression.

- Mental health disorders are defined in imprecise ways. There is not a clear line between normal behavioural variation and behavioural disorders.

- The biggest indicator of whether you should consider seeking help for your child is whether their behaviour is causing impairment; in other words, is their behaviour causing challenges at home, with peers, or at school?

- The sooner you seek help for your child's behavioural or emotional challenges, the sooner your child can start learning skills to overcome them. So don't wait! Many child behavioural and emotional problems get worse over time if left untreated.

CHAPTER 9

Putting It All Together:
A New Approach to Parenting

I t's a running joke in my family that I have spent more time in the head teacher's office since I had children than I ever did in the twenty-plus years that I was actually a student. That certainly wasn't part of my imagined life plan, coming from my experience as a straight-A student with multiple degrees in psychology. So if your children are not quite turning out to be the people you imagined raising, you're not alone. Mine aren't perfect, and I'm considered an "expert" in child behaviour (my husband still finds that hilarious).

The reality is that as a parent you are only responsible for doing your best. *You are not responsible for your child's behaviour.* Wait, what? Not responsible for my child's behaviour? That feels counterintuitive. But anyone who has ever tried to buckle a squirming toddler into a car seat has realised that it is very hard to *make* anyone do anything—no matter their size.

It's your job to help and to teach your child. But it's your *child's* job to implement these lessons. So be kind to yourself, and to fellow parents. It's hard to accept, but much of our children's behaviour is ultimately out of our control. We can guide and shape them, but we cannot control them. In the end, how they behave and who they become is their choice.

It's a fact that we will have to remind ourselves of over and over again as they grow up and we slip back into our "parental moulding" role, forgetting how much control our own children have over their destiny.

Let's imagine for a second what parenting looks like in a world where we have all internalised that basic fact—that as parents we are not in control of our children's behaviour. In that world, we do our best with our children, but we don't feel immense guilt when they are having a tantrum in a shop. We don't feel the weight of judgement from others as our child sulks in the corner at the birthday party. We support one another as parents. We exchange ideas, but we recognise that every child is different. We marvel and laugh with other parents in the playgroup when one parent tries implementing another's "magic" behaviour chart and it completely backfires in their child—*and we don't assume that parent must have been doing something wrong*. We present our parenting ideas as suggestions, not as gospel, recognising that what works for one child may not work for another child—including their sibling! We recognise that when we get "easy", well-behaved children, we lucked out—that their behaviour is as much about their temperament as it is about our excellent parenting. We empathise with parents who have challenging children and recognise that their little genetic roll of the dice is giving them a run for their money. Rather than judging them, we support parents whose kiddos are acting out, or struggling.

If this world feels unrealistic, it's only because we've allowed Freud, and our mothers, and all those other "experts" who have produced cottage industries telling parents what they should be doing, to dominate our narrative. In the same way that we have evolved with the science and changed our views on what causes autism (no, it's not caused by cold mothers), it's time to change the way we view all of child behaviour, and stop blaming parents when kids aren't perfect. It's not bad parenting that's causing our kids to misbehave. They're just kids. And some kids are naturally disposed to be more impulsive, more emotional, more defiant, and more frustrating than others. By embracing the science behind children's individual differences, we can create a more supportive, less judgemental culture of parenting.

In the child development literature, there is the concept of "good enough" parenting. The idea is that, as parents, we don't have to follow a precise plan for our children to turn out OK. Our super-parenting isn't going to shape them into super-beings. You cannot feed a child whose genes predispose them to be short more and more food such that they grow to be six feet tall. Conversely, you *can* malnourish a child such that they don't reach their full stature. But as long as the environment is within a normal range, our kids will grow up to be their own people based in large part on their unique genetic codes. Our job is just to do "good enough" so that they have the chance to blossom.

To be clear, good enough parenting does *not* mean that what we do as parents is not important. Parents are important in critical ways—*but it's just not the ways most of us spend our time worrying about*. It's not in whether we allow a pacifier, or how we potty train, or the exact amount of screen time we allow that will determine the people our children will become. (Though it's probably not a good idea to sit them in front of the TV all day every day.) Remember: our children already have genetic codes that are programmed to grow them into full-fledged human beings, with all the dizzying and amazing array of characteristics that come along with being human. Despite what the media, our parents, and our parent-friends tell us, *the vast majority of things we agonise over as parents are just not that important for the big picture of how our kids will turn out*. Their genes are doing the heavy lifting.

There are still lots of ways we can be great parents—that we can do better than "good enough". Being a great parent starts with recognising who your child is by genetic design. By accepting and loving that child, you can help them grow into their best possible self, recognising that person may not be the person you originally imagined your child would be.

Understanding your child's unique code can help you flexibly adapt your parenting to help them grow into the best version of themselves; you can help them appreciate and accentuate their strengths, and work with them on their challenges. By understanding what pieces you have control over, and what pieces you don't, you can use that knowledge to help your child reach their potential. Challenges come when you try to "change" your child. If you spend all your time talking about how much you want them to be tall, and trying to force-feed them, you're only going to make a child genetically predisposed to be short feel bad about themselves. That seems obvious when it comes to height, but it's true of behaviour as well.

Hopefully at this point you are feeling empowered! You have science on your side. You have a better understanding of your child, and how their unique genetic code shapes their development. You understand how your genotype influences your temperament, your tendencies, and the way you interact with your child. You feel less pressured because you know there is no such thing as a perfect way to parent. You can flexibly adapt your parenting to your child, reducing frustrations and stress points, and focusing on what matters most for each individual. You can know that you're doing your best, but you are ultimately not in control of, or responsible for, your child's behaviour and outcomes. You know what signs to look out for, and you know when to seek help.

But maybe you're feeling overwhelmed. Maybe the idea that you have less control over your child's behaviour and life outcomes is frightening, or leaves you feeling disheartened if your child is struggling. Maybe it's causing you to question why you are spending so much time and energy focused on your child if you don't have the ability to shape them in the way you might have imagined.

If you are feeling that way, imagine for a second you're talking about a spouse or a close friend instead of your child. You probably also invest in spending a lot of time with them, but presumably you're spending time with that person because you love them and want to build a relationship with them. You are not spending time with them because you are trying to change them or mould them into the person you want them to be. If you're happily married (or even still married), you likely abandoned that idea some time ago, and you have learned to work through frustration points and build a relationship that takes into account each of your individual needs, desires, and personalities. It's true of close, lasting friendships as well.

Just like your partner, or your best friend, your child is their own person. A smaller person, to be sure, and one who needs you to help them grow into themselves. But they too are their own unique person—a person that you will get to know, and who will have things about them you love, and things about them that are, ahem, not your favourite. Just like the other people in your life who you love, your child is a person with whom you have the opportunity to build a relationship; the quality and nature of that relationship will depend a lot on whether you accept them and love them for the person that they are.

Good parenting is not a matter of just doing more. It's a matter of figuring out what's right for your child—for their unique genetic code—as it unfolds across all their developmental stages. Child development is characterised by both stability and change. Genetic influences largely contribute to what is stable across development, but the way those dispositions unfold and get expressed at different ages will evolve. It will shift depending on how you nudge them in one direction or another, and many other aspects of their environment. It will change depending on their experiences with peers, their teachers, their coaches, and other life events—some of which you can influence, and some of which you can't.

For me, one of the hardest parts of being a parent is acknowledging, and learning to accept and live with, the vast array of things that are out of my control when it comes to my children. When my friends and I were in our twenties, before any of us had children, we all had grand ideas about how we were going to throw our kids in backpacks and keep right on hiking, camping, and travelling the world (I lived in Alaska back then). For some of us, it worked. Others ended up stuck at home with colicky babies, or small toddlers who threw massive tantrums that made travelling impossible, or children who had developmental disabilities.

Trying to control the way things turn out with children ignores basic facts about the nature of human behaviour. It just leads to frustration, for you and your child. At worst, trying too hard to shape your child can actually stand in the way of allowing them to grow, and it can damage your relationship with them. Ultimately, children need to learn how to manage their own temperaments and tendencies. One of the best things you can do as a parent is to help them with that process. This includes allowing them to experience the good, and the bad, that come from making different decisions. If they don't have the opportunity to try and fail, then they won't learn how to do better in the future.

As a parent, you can be there to support and encourage your child as they go through that growth process. The older they get, the more weight and potential consequences their decisions hold, so they need to start practising from the time they are young. As much as we love our children, we can't always be there for them. Nor should we be. Perhaps in the end, the greatest gift we can give our children is to let go enough to allow them to become their own person; to let their unique genetic code sing; to realise that their song may be different from our own; and to enjoy the concert anyway, even when it's not the one we expected to be attending.

BUT WAIT, THERE'S MORE!

Parents, our journey together doesn't end here. Join me at my website **danielledick.com**, where you will find additional resources, information, and support for raising your unique little bundle of genes.

ACKNOWLEDGEMENTS

I am incredibly grateful to the many people who made this book possible.

To my colleague Everett Worthington, who was the first person to talk with me about the nuts and bolts of writing a trade book. Thank you for being generous with your time, sharing your materials, and starting me on this journey.

To my agent, Carolyn Savarese. You took my nugget of an idea and turned it into this book! Thank you for seeing my vision, helping me shape it, getting others to see the potential in it, and being my champion through the whole process. I am indebted to you for making my dream a reality.

To my editor, Lucia Watson, and the whole team at Avery and Penguin Random House. You made this process fun and smooth! I look forward to the adventure ahead. Thank you, Lucia, for believing in me and helping this book become its best.

To my parents, Dan and Lynn Dick. Thank you for your constant love, for always believing in me and encouraging me to follow my dreams, for being tireless champions. You have always been the first to celebrate my accomplishments, and to be there when things don't turn out as planned too. I wish everyone were lucky enough to have parents like you.

To my husband, Casey, who has enriched my life in so many ways, including by bringing my beautiful stepdaughter, Nora, into it. You had the vision for what this book would become long before I did. Thank you for your kind heart, patience, and support, for being a wonderful husband and father, for challenging me to expand my thinking (even when I don't want to hear it, which is usually), for being my effusive champion, and for bringing such joy into my life.

To my beautiful children, Aidan and Nora, who are so different and special in their own ways. I can't wait to see where your unique journeys take you. Aidan, I thought I knew everything there was to know about parenting until I had you! Thank you for making me a mum, for your patience when I have fallen short, and for sharing this journey with me. I am so proud of how far you have come, and the person you are growing up to be.

To my siblings, Jeanine and Bryan, who have been along for the ride on all of my adventures, and their spouses, John and April, for rounding out our close family. I love sharing the craziness of raising small people with strong Dick family genes with all of you.

To the family I inherited, my mother- and sister-in-law, Susan and Barbara, thank you for being engaged and excited about *all* of my projects with me. I hit the jackpot when I married Casey and got you as my bonus family.

To the many friends who have enriched my parenting journey. I will not attempt to list you all here for fear of leaving anyone off the list—you know who you are. Thank you for sharing your stories and listening to mine, for being a source of joy and support. Parenting is so much more fun when you can share the good, the bad, and the ugly with your friends! Thank you especially to Gretchen Winterstein, who provided constructive feedback on early chapters of this book, and who has been a steadfast friend through so many life stages, dating back to our chance meeting the first week of college. Thank you as well to my dear friend Stephanie Davis Michelman, who allowed me to share some of her parenting stories in the book.

Thank you to my first mentors in behaviour genetics, the late Irving Gottesman, my undergraduate adviser who introduced me to the field, and Richard Rose, my graduate adviser. Both had an incalculable effect on my life and I am forever grateful. Thank you to my colleague, friend, and fellow parent Jessica Salvatore, who read an early version of this book and was kind enough to let me include stories about her own parenting journey. To my EDGE (Examining Development, Genes, and Environment) lab team: thank you for listening to endless stories about my children, and for indulging my never-ending passion for trying new things. I am also indebted to all the researchers who spend their lives generating knowledge. We are a product of our histories, and mine is shaped by the hundreds of scholars who have come before me to generate the research that has shaped my thinking, my parenting, and, accordingly, this book. Please know that this book is a tribute to all your hard work, even though it deviates from our typical scholarly output.

Finally, to my dear friend Marshall Lynch. Where do I start? You have contributed so much to this book that you probably deserve a by-line! I know you will recognise your influence throughout, honed from our Saturday morning coffee dates, pandemic video chats, and countless hours of conversation about our children and lives. Thank you for reading every chapter of every draft, and for being my partner on this project every step of the way. You elevate everything and everyone in your life; this book benefited tremendously by being in your orbit. I am so grateful for your friendship.

To you, my reader, in the trenches raising your own unique small person. I see you. I know what it's like when your little "bundle of joy" is giving you a run for your money. Thank you for reading through to the end; this book is for you.

RESOURCES AND RECOMMENDED READING

As I noted at the beginning, this book is intended to be a user-friendly guide for parents, rather than a scholarly review of the literature. Here I provide recommendations for books that provide more information about the research covered in *The Child Code*, as well as additional parenting books that I have found helpful.

Temperament

If you are looking for a scholarly review of research on temperament, I highly recommend *Becoming Who We Are: Temperament and Personality in Development* (Guilford Press, 2012) by Mary K. Rothbart. Dr Rothbart, a retired distinguished professor, is one of the world's leading experts on temperament. This book provides an in-depth review of the large literature on temperament, including many of the studies that are mentioned in this book. There is also an extensive scientific reference section.

Temperament in the Classroom: Understanding Individual Differences (Paul H. Brookes Publishing Company, 2002), edited by Barbara K. Keogh, Ph.D., does a really nice job of reviewing the temperament literature, and goes into greater detail about the research behind how temperament plays out in the school setting.

Behaviour Genetics

If you're looking for an academic book that provides further information about methods and findings from the field of behaviour genetics, I recommend *Behavioural Genetics*, seventh edition (Worth Publishers, Macmillan Learning, 2017), a comprehensive textbook by Valerie S. Knopik, Jenae M. Neiderhiser, John C. DeFries, and Robert Plomin.

If you're looking for a more user-friendly read geared towards general audiences, I recommend Robert Plomin's *Blueprint: How DNA Makes Us Who We Are* (MIT Press, 2018).

Parenting Books

Here is a selection of my favourite parenting books, ones that are evidence-based and that have helped me in my parenting journey. Parents of High Em children may especially benefit from some of these in-depth books on parenting strategies.

1-2-3 Magic: The New Three-Step Discipline for Calm, Effective, and Happy Parenting, sixth edition (Sourcebooks, 2016) by Thomas W. Phelan, Ph.D.

The Explosive Child: A New Approach for Understanding and Parenting Easily Frustrated, Chronically Inflexible Children (HarperCollins, 2005) by Ross W. Greene, Ph.D.

Freeing Your Child from Anxiety: Powerful Strategies to Overcome Fears, Worries, and Phobias, revised edition (Harmony Books, 2014) by Tamar E. Chansky, Ph.D.

The Kazdin Method for Parenting the Defiant Child: With No Pills, No Therapy, No Contest of Wills (Mariner Books, 2009) by Alan E. Kazdin, Ph.D., director of the Yale Parenting Center and Child Conduct Clinic.

Parenting the Strong-Willed Child: The Clinically Proven Five-Week Program for Parents of Two- to Six-Year-Olds, updated edition (McGraw Hill, 2002) by Rex Forehand, Ph.D., and Nicholas Long, Ph.D.

NOTES

INTRODUCTION: Understanding the Child Code

5 **Developmental psychologists refer:** M. K. Rothbart and J. E. Bates, "Temperament," in W. Damon and N. Eisenberg, eds, *Handbook of Child Psychology: Social, Emotional, and Personality Development*, 5th edn, vol. 3 (New York, NY: John Wiley and Sons, 1998), 105–76.

8 **This is called *precision medicine*:** F. S. Collins and H. Varmus, "A New Initiative on Precision Medicine," *New England Journal of Medicine* 372, no. 9 (2015): 793–95.

CHAPTER 1: Nature Versus Nurture: The Science Is In

21 **followed nearly 1,300 children:** J. Lansford et al., "Bidirectional Relations between Parenting and Behaviour Problems from Age 8 to 13 in Nine Countries," *Journal of Research on Adolescence* 28, no. 3 (2018): 571–90.

24 **In the late 1960s, a researcher published:** L. L. Heston, "Psychiatric Disorders in Foster Home Reared Children of Schizophrenic Mothers," *British Journal of Psychiatry* 112 (1966): 819–25.

25 **We now know that schizophrenia:** P. Sullivan, K. S. Kendler, and M. C. Neale, "Schizophrenia as a Complex Trait: Evidence from a Meta-analysis of Twin Studies," *Archives of General Psychiatry* 60, no. 12 (2003): 1187–92.

25 **ranging from alcohol problems:** K. S. Kendler et al., "An Extended Swedish National Adoption Study of Alcohol Use Disorder," *JAMA Psychiatry* 72, no. 3 (2015): 211–18.

25 **infant shyness:** D. Daniels and R. Plomin, "Origins of Individual Differences in Infant Shyness," *Developmental Psychology* 21, no. 1 (1985): 118–21.

25 **Adoption studies have also been pivotal:** R. J. Cadoret, "Adoption Studies," *Alcohol Health and Research World* 19, no. 3 (1995): 195–200.

25 **a Swedish adoption study examined criminal behaviour:** K. S. Kendler et al., "A Swedish National Adoption Study of Criminality," *Psychological Medicine* 44, no. 9 (2014): 1913–25.

29 **Many countries have national twin registries:** Y.-M. Hur and J. M. Craig, "Twin Registries Worldwide: An Important Resource for Scientific Research," *Twin Research and Human Genetics* 16, no. 1 (2013): 1–12.

29 **I work on a study:** R. J. Rose et al., "FinnTwin12 Cohort: An Updated Review," *Twin Research and Human Genetics* 22, no. 5 (2019): 302–11; M. Kaidesoja et al., "Finn-Twin16: A Longitudinal Study from Age 16 of a Population-based Finnish Twin Cohort," *Twin Research and Human Genetics* 22, no. 6 (2019): 530–39.

29 **a large twin registry in the Netherlands:** L. Lighart et al., "The Netherlands Twin Register: Longitudinal Research Based on Twin and Twin-family Designs," *Twin Research and Human Genetics* 22, no. 6 (2019): 623–36.

29 **My current university is home:** E. C. H. Lilley, A.-T. Morris, and J. L. Silberg, "The Mid-Atlantic Twin Registry of Virginia Commonwealth University," *Twin Research and Human Genetics* 22, no. 6 (2019): 753–56.

30 **Studies of substance use and psychiatric disorders:** K. S. Kendler, C. A. Prescott, J. Myers, and M. C. Neale, "The Structure of Genetic and Environmental Risk Factors for Common Psychiatric and Substance Use Disorders in Men and Women," *Archives of General Psychiatry* 60, no. 9 (2003): 929–37.

30 **personality and intelligence:** T. J. Bouchard Jr. and M. McGue, "Genetic and Environmental Influences on Human Psychological Differences," *Journal of Neurobiology* 54 (2003): 4–45.

30 **studies of divorce:** M. McGue and D. T. Lykken, "Genetic Influence on Risk of Divorce," *Psychological Science* 3, no. 6 (1992): 368–73.

30 **happiness:** M. Bartels and D. I. Boomsma, "Born to Be Happy? The Etiology of Subjective Well-being," *Behaviour Genetics* 39, no. 6 (2009): 605–15.

30 **voting behaviour:** P. K. Hatemi et al., "The Genetics of Voting: An Australian Twin Study," *Behaviour Genetics* 37, no. 3 (2007): 435–48.

30 **religiosity:** T. Vance, H. H. Maes, and K. S. Kendler, "Genetic and Environmental Influences on Multiple Dimensions of Religiosity: A Twin Study," *Journal of Nervous and Mental Disease* 198, no. 10 (2010): 755–61.

30 **social attitudes, and almost anything else:** L. Eaves et al., "Comparing the Biological and Cultural Inheritance of Personality and Social Attitudes in the Virginia 30,000 Study of Twins and their Relatives," *Twin Research* 2 (1999): 62–80.

30 **A huge study of self-control:** Y. E. Willems et al., "The Heritability of Self-Control: A Meta-analysis," *Neuroscience Biobehavioural Review* 100 (2019): 324–34.

30 **Anxiety/depression in three-year-olds:** D. I. Boomsma et al., "Genetic and Environmental Influences on Anxious/Depression during Childhood: A Study from the Netherlands Twin Register," *Genes, Brain and Behaviour* 4 (2005): 466–81.

30 **Behaviour problems in seven-year-olds:** B. C. Haberstick et al., "Contributions of Genes and Environments to Stability and Change in Externalizing and Internalizing Problems during Elementary and Middle School," *Behaviour Genetics* 35, no. 4 (2005): 381–96.

31 **"All human behavioural traits are heritable":** E. Turkheimer, "Three Laws of Behaviour Genetics and What They Mean," *Current Directions in Psychological Science* 9, no. 5 (2000): 160–64.

32 **in the late 1970s, researchers from the University of Minnesota:** Nancy Segal, *Born Together–Reared Apart: The Landmark Minnesota Twin Study* (Cambridge, MA: Harvard University Press, 2012); see also: https://mctfr.psych.umn.edu/research/UM%20research.html.

CHAPTER 2: It's Complicated: The Ways That Genes Influence Our Lives

35 **One of my favourite articles:** R. Sapolsky, "A Gene for Nothing," *Discover* magazine, September 30, 1997.

37 **more at risk of developing alcohol problems:** H. Begleiter et al., "The Collaborative Study on the Genetics of Alcoholism," *Alcohol and Health Research World* 19 (1995): 228–36.

38 **intertwining of our genetic predispositions:** S. Scarr and K. McCartney, "How People Make Their Own Environments: A Theory of Genotype Greater than Environment Effects," *Child Development* 54, no. 2 (1983): 424–35.

45 **We know that intelligence is heritable:** R. Plomin and S. von Stumm, (2018). "The New Genetics of Intelligence," *Nature Reviews Genetics* 19, no. 3 (2018): 148–59.

45 **we know that aggression is significantly genetically influenced:** C. Tuvblad and L. A. Baker, "Human Aggression across the Lifespan: Genetic Propensities and Environmental Moderators," *Advances in Genetics* 75 (2011): 171–214.

47 **We call this *gene-environment interaction*:** D. M. Dick, "Gene-environment Interaction in Psychological Traits and Disorders," *Annual Review of Clinical Psychology* 7 (2011): 383–409.

CHAPTER 3: Getting to Know Your Child: "The Big Three" Dimensions of Temperament

64 **In child development, we call this *Goodness of Fit*:** S. Chess and A. Thomas, *Goodness of Fit: Clinical Applications for Infancy through Adult Life* (Philadelphia: Bruner/Mazel, 1999).

68 **Psychologist Carol Dweck has written extensively:** Carol S. Dweck, Ph.D., *Mindset: The New Psychology of Success* (New York: Ballantine Books, 2007).

CHAPTER 4: Extraversion: The "Ex" Factor

90 **one unexpected way extraverts may get an edge:** K. A. Duffy and T. L. Chartrand, "The Extravert Advantage: How and When Extraverts Build Rapport with Other People," *Psychological Science* 26, no. 11 (2015): 1795–802.

CHAPTER 6: Effortful Control: The "Ef" Factor

157 **came to be known as the Marshmallow Test:** Walter Mischel, *The Marshmallow Test: Why Self-Control Is the Engine of Success* (Boston: Little, Brown, 2015).

158 **longitudinal study conducted in New Zealand:** T. E. Moffitt et al., "A Gradient of Childhood Self-control Predicts Health, Wealth, and Public Safety," *Proceedings of the National Academy of Sciences of the United States* 108 (2011): 2693–98.

CHAPTER 7: Beyond You and Your Child: Predispositions and Partners

192 **he reviewed more than 250 samples:** T. M. Achenbach, S. H. McConaughy, and C. T. Howell, "Child/Adolescent Behavioural and Emotional Problems: Implications of Cross-informant Correlations for Situational Specificity," *Psychological Bulletin* 101, no. 2 (1987): 213–32.

CHAPTER 9: Putting It All Together: A New Approach to Parenting

235 **concept of "good enough" parenting:** S. Scarr, "Developmental Theories for the 1990s: Development and Individual Differences," *Child Development* 63, no. 1 (1992): 1–19.

INDEX

Page numbers in bold indicate tables, those in italics indicate figures; those followed by "n" indicate notes.